ABOUTFACE

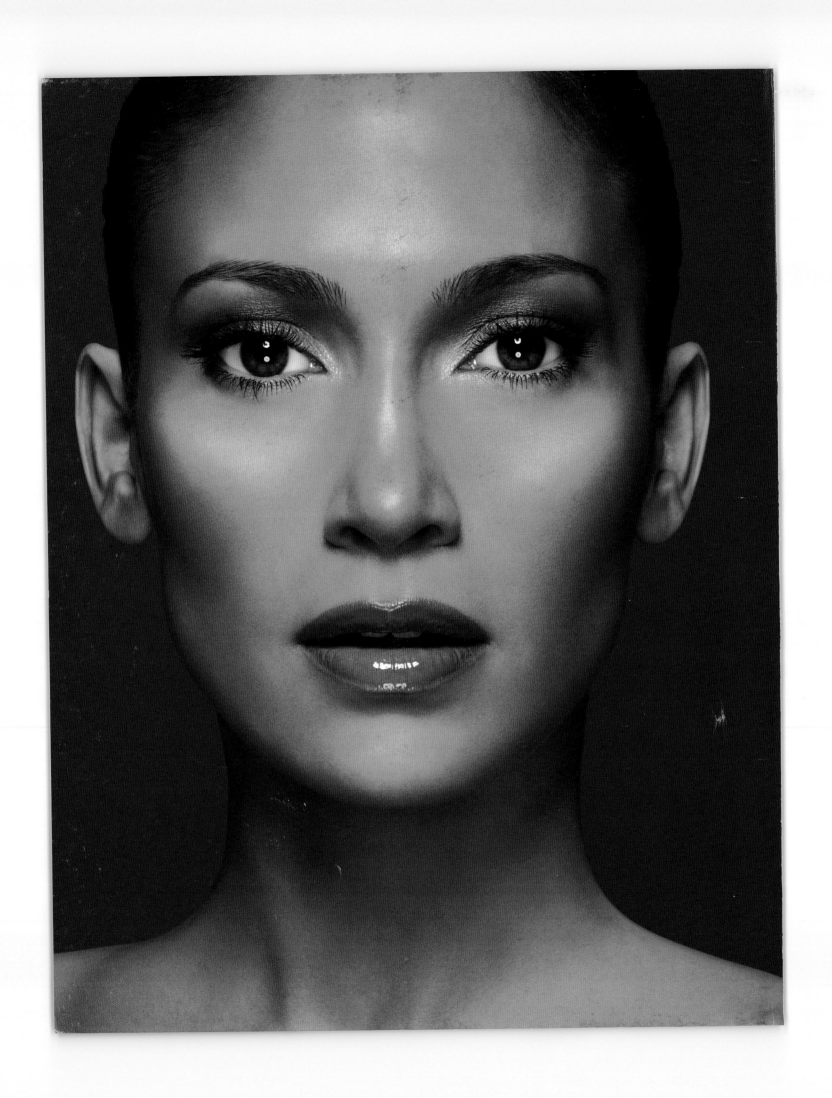

SCOTTBARNES

ABOUTFACE

AMAZING TRANSFORMATIONS USING THE SECRETS OF THE TOP CELEBRITY MAKEUP ARTIST

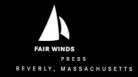

FAIR WINDS
PRESS
BEVERLY, MASSACHUSETTS

Text © 2010 Scott Barnes

First published in the USA in 2010 by
Fair Winds Press, a member of
Quayside Publishing Group
100 Cummings Center
Suite 406-L
Beverly, MA 01915-6101
www.fairwindspress.com

14 13 12 11 10   2 3 4 5

ISBN-13: 978-1-59233-399-8
ISBN-10: 1-59233-399-0

Library of Congress Cataloging-in-Publication Data
Barnes, Scott, 1968-
  About face : amazing transformations using the secrets of the top celebrity makeup
artist / Scott Barnes.
     p. cm.
  ISBN-13: 978-1-59233-399-8
  ISBN-10: 1-59233-399-0
 1. Beauty, Personal. 2. Beauty culture. 3. Cosmetics. 4. Celebrities--Miscellanea. I.
Title.
  RA778.B2295 2010
  646.7'26--dc22

                                                        2009031147

Cover and book design by Alisha Neumaier
Book layout by Carol Holtz
Photography by Karl Simone

PRINTED AND BOUND IN CHINA

In memory
   of my brother,
John Barnes.

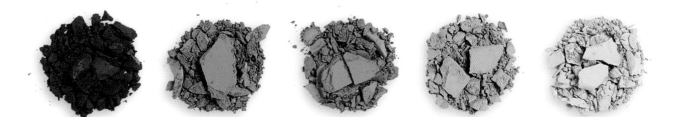

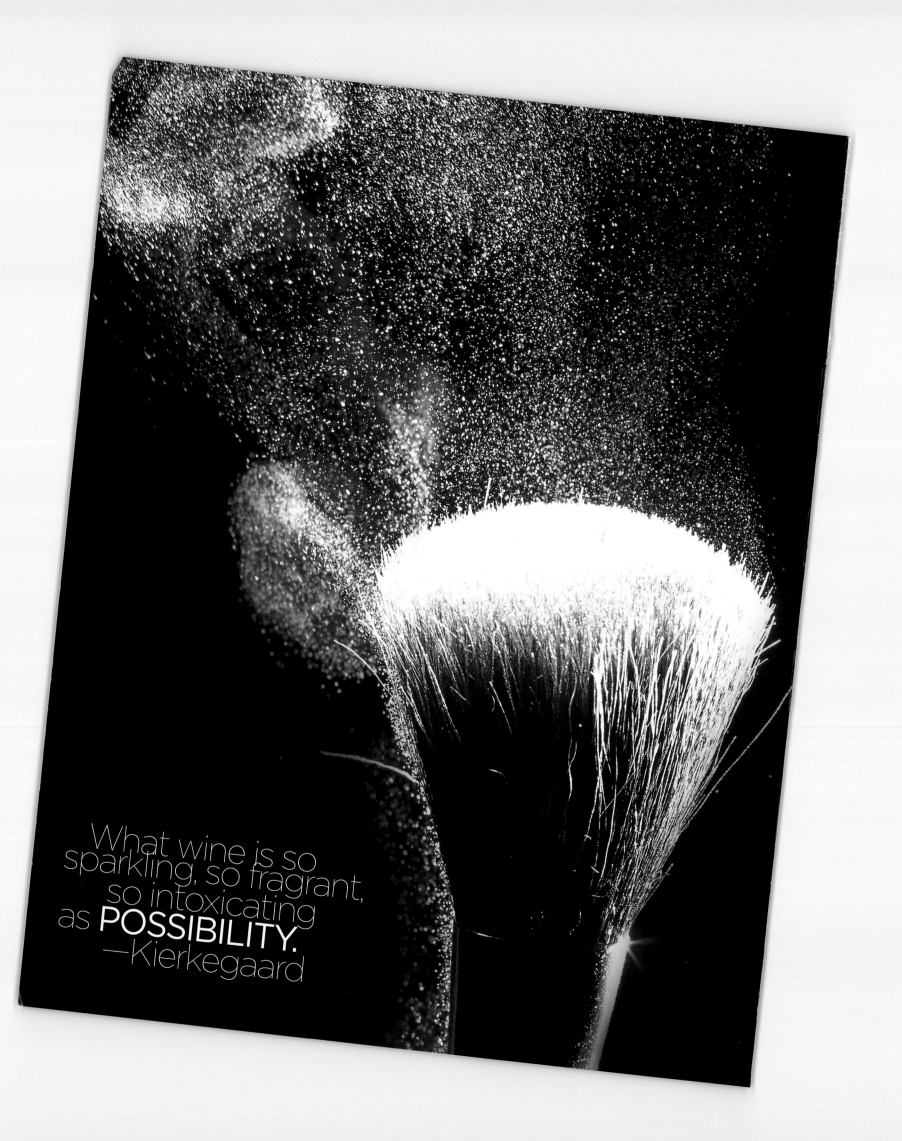

What wine is so sparkling, so fragrant, so intoxicating as POSSIBILITY.
—Kierkegaard

contents

foreword

It was springtime or summer of 2000 or 2001.
I can't remember exactly, but I do remember the
sun was shining. It was a beautiful day. I was doing
a photo shoot for *In Style* magazine in downtown
Manhattan, and I was trying out a new makeup
artist, which can always be interesting...

I walked over to the hair and makeup table and
a guy with a big smile and a head full of cherubic,
light brown curls held out his hand to me and said,
"Hi, I'm Scott," and I immediately felt at home.
I don't know if it was the warmth of his smile or
the easy, comfortable way about him, but
I knew it was going to be a special day!

I sat down in the chair and immediately Scott
went to work. He said, "I am all about skin, and
yours is gorgeous. We are gonna make you glow!!"
Well, I didn't realize the half of it. His lovely, positive
attitude and personality were only a precursor to
his talent, which can be described as nothing
short of makeup magic. He had a special touch.
Long story short, he has been making me "glow"
ever since!

That same day I told him I had another photo shoot
and a video shoot coming up for my new album,
J.Lo, and I told him, "I want you to do it." We started
talking about ideas and realized we had a lot in
common. One thing we shared was that we both
love glamour and anything glamorous, and since
that sunny afternoon we have created a countless
number of glamorous moments together. And
that's where it was born: a relationship that
continues to this day.

One of the many blessings of working in this
business is getting to work with other artists
who have a passion for what they do. From that
passion, they are able to change the future and
create what's new and what's modern—what's
today. This is the kind of talent Scott has. He's a
true artist. He wants everyone to be beautiful and
feel beautiful inside and out, and he has always
made me feel that way when I am sitting in his
chair: that I am the most beautiful woman in the
world (and trust me: that is no easy task on a
movie set at 5:30 in the morning).

Like any relationship that spans years we have
been through so much together: ups and
downs, ins and outs. We have worked through
disagreements, breakups, marriages, divorces,
and even deaths, growing closer through it all as
true friends do. I am honored to have been able
to work with this man who I believe to be the best
makeup artist in the business today. But I am even
more honored to call him my dear, dear friend.
I hope you enjoy this book and all of its helpful
information and little secrets, many of which he
has used on this face, too!!

Have an absolutely beautiful time!
I know you will.

love
jennifer

Photograph by Marc Anthony.

introduction

Transformation

It's a powerful concept, especially when it comes to your appearance. And *About Face* is about the ability to transform your look from average to extraordinary. Makeup can certainly work to transform a person. It can help a woman feel more confident, sexy, and beautiful. But this book isn't just about makeup techniques. It's about learning how to accept yourself and enhance what you've got. You have to feel good about yourself before you can begin to feel beautiful. You've heard the old cliché, "Beauty starts from within." Like it or not, ladies, it's a true statement.

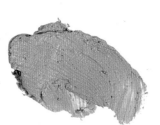

Most of us look in the mirror and focus on what we wish we could change. My forehead is too high, my lips are too thin, or my cheeks are too fat...the list goes on. But what if you looked in the mirror and focused on the fact that all these things you don't like about yourself are the very things that make you you? That's your uniqueness, what sets you apart. Finding your beauty isn't about looking exactly like everyone else. It's about accepting yourself—the parts you love and the parts you don't—and then working with all of it.

When I look at women I find each and every one of them beautiful. Because each and every woman is distinct. The combination of face shape, features, and smile: that's what makes a woman beautiful. All the women in this book started out gorgeous in their own way, and I simply gave them new ways to emphasize their unparalleled look. So, as you read about the various makeup techniques I present here and check out the transformations, take a look at yourself in the mirror and remind yourself that, among the millions of women out there, there's no one quite like you. Be gentle with yourself. Love yourself. Embrace the beauty of "you." Once you've done that, you're ready to start playing with the power of makeup to transform yourself into anything you want to be, including your most beautiful, most exceptional self.

About Face contains beauty rituals I've perfected over my years of working with many models and celebrities, as well as expert advice from my team of trusted consultants. You'll find portraits, step-by-step guides, and interviews with many women describing their own beauty regimens and transformations. You can use this information to affect your own transformation, capitalizing on

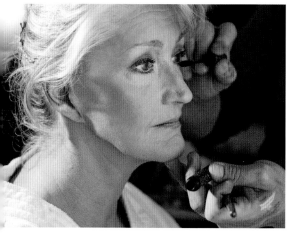

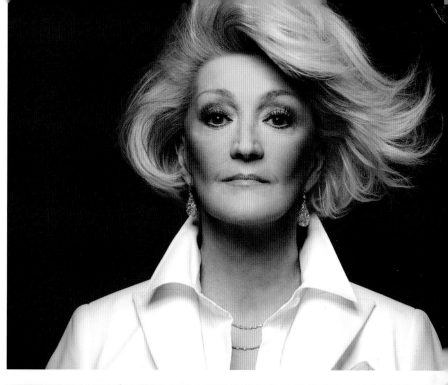

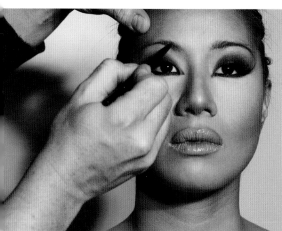

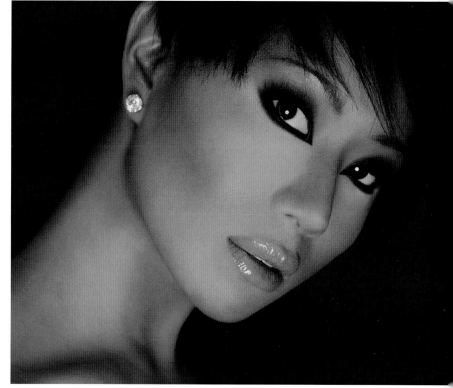

your distinct features to create a look that's unequaled. I want all women, not just my clients, to feel beautiful and empowered. Feeling beautiful leads to self-respect. Self-respect leads to greater confidence. And confidence commands attention. So, let's begin your journey to becoming your most beautiful, most exceptional self.

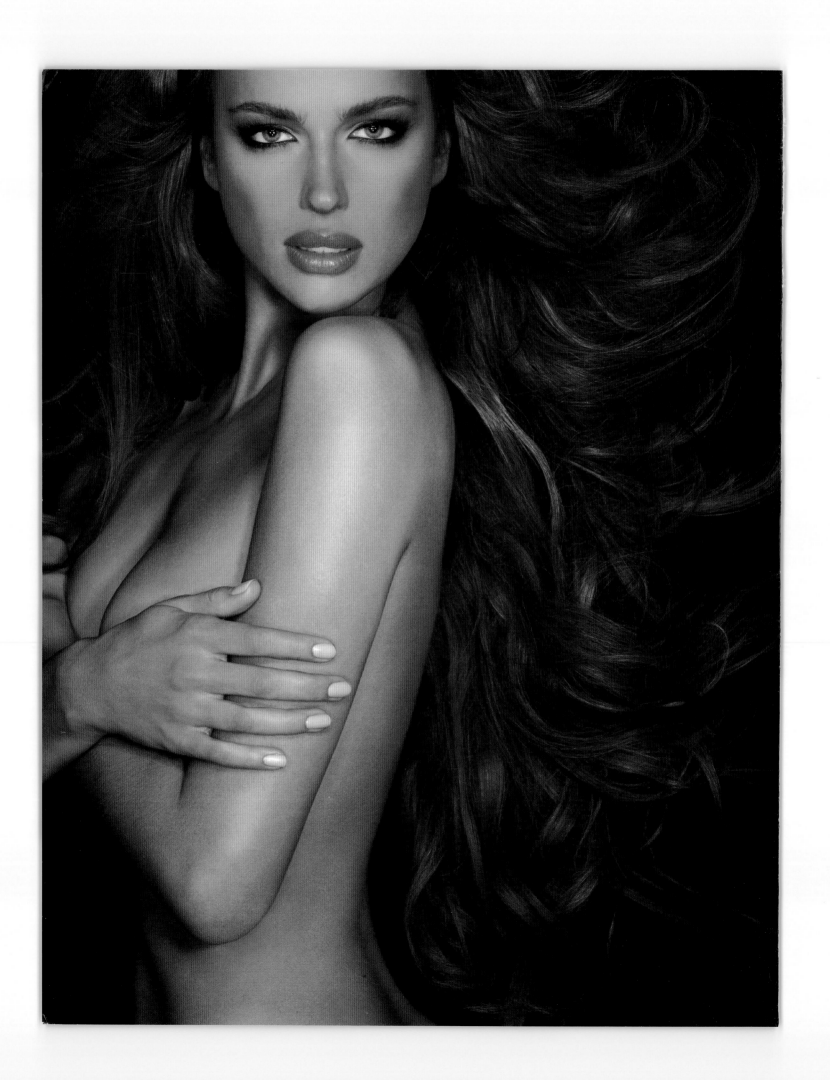

THE GLAM SQUAD

Karl Simone
(PHOTORAPHY)

I was born and raised in Toronto. I first picked up a camera in high school art class, fell in love with it, and never really put it down. I have always found it necessary to be creative. It's just something that comes naturally to me, and I am so appreciative that I get to do something creative for a living. I met Scott in Miami in the early 1990s, and he and I immediately hit it off. We both share a love for creating something beautiful and have been talking about shooting a book together for a while. I am extremely proud of what we have created, our collaboration on these images, and our friendship.

They say "Beauty is in the eye of the beholder," but as I've learned through my experience as a photographer, it is also in the beholder of the camera.

The camera is a very strange instrument. It allows people to take on a new identity. It's about photographing not only those who are beautiful but also those who feel beautiful. Creating an "illusion" of beauty begins with a process. Makeup, hair, clothing, and lighting—each is an essential ingredient, but they are not as important as a woman's sense of self. These women were on a journey that took them to another level of self-awareness that translated on both sides of the lens. Each is unique in personality, yet they all share the same desire to feel great about who they are as women.

Watching Scott transform them, I saw their faces change both physically and emotionally. It was amazing and inspiring to witness, to say the least. As each woman stepped in front of the camera, I was able to capture a new-found confidence and beauty. This was, indeed, a transformational experience for each and every one of them. After all, it is about face.

Chuck Amos (HAIR)

I love working with hair and making women feel beautiful. You must feel beautiful to be beautiful. If you really like a particular look, even if other people say it looks crazy on you, that's what you should go for. Because it shines through who you are, you feel comfortable and great. Being beautiful on the outside is really just an enhancement to what you can feel on the inside. There's no real standard of beauty. I think it's different for each person.

I never want to overtake my clients' look by giving them over-the-top hair if they feel uncomfortable about it; yet, I want to give the world something they've never seen in hair before. I see myself more as a hair artist/illusionist than a hairstylist because my learning journey on the subject has been from every aspect. So, now I can do or make just about anything with hair, from major sculptures to organizing fashion show hair for twenty-five models. There is nothing I cannot do with hair at this point, and I love the adventure of it. The passion for it overtakes the feeling of work, so it's easy to put all my heart into my work. I've touched the heads of Diana Ross, Donna Summer, En Vogue, Beyoncé, Destiny's Child, Vanessa Williams, Tyra Banks, Naomi Campbell, Lauren Hutton, Ivana Trump, Jewel... the list goes on. In addition to working with many wonderful celebrities, some of the highlights of my career include doing a Versace show in South Africa (and meeting Nelson Mandela) and being the first African American to do the hair for the cover of *Paris Vogue*.

Ultimately, I like to consider myself an illusionist instead of a hairstylist since I do all sorts of tricks with hair that no one usually sees. (I was doing extensions when they were considered faux pas!) Scott is the face and body illusionist; he showed me how the illusion of makeup can really work with the illusion of hair. The end result is true genius.

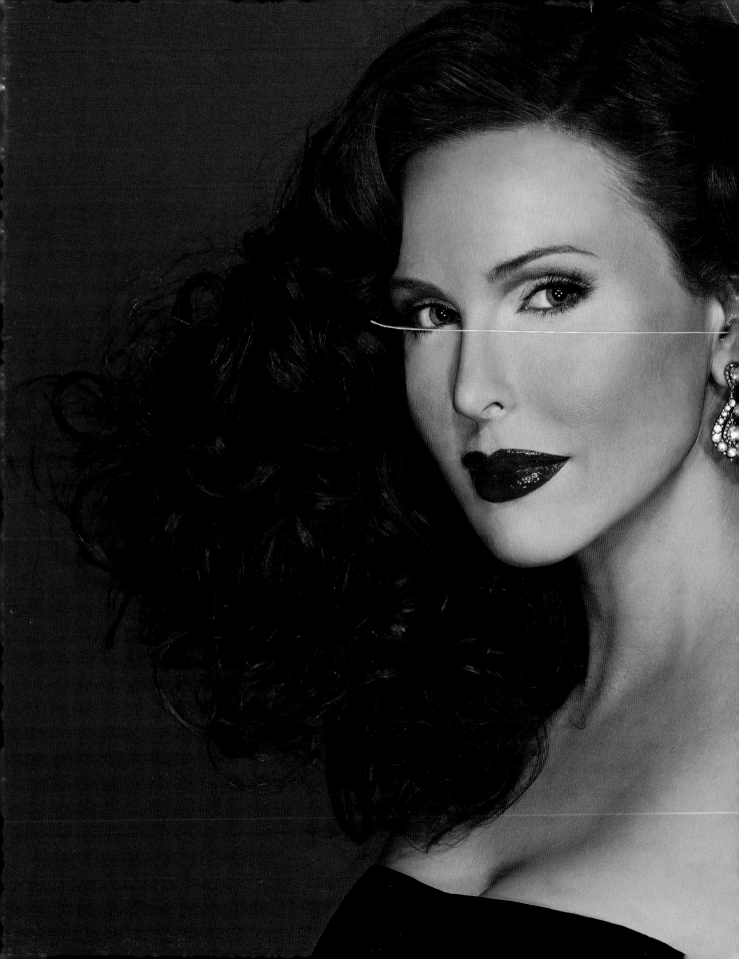

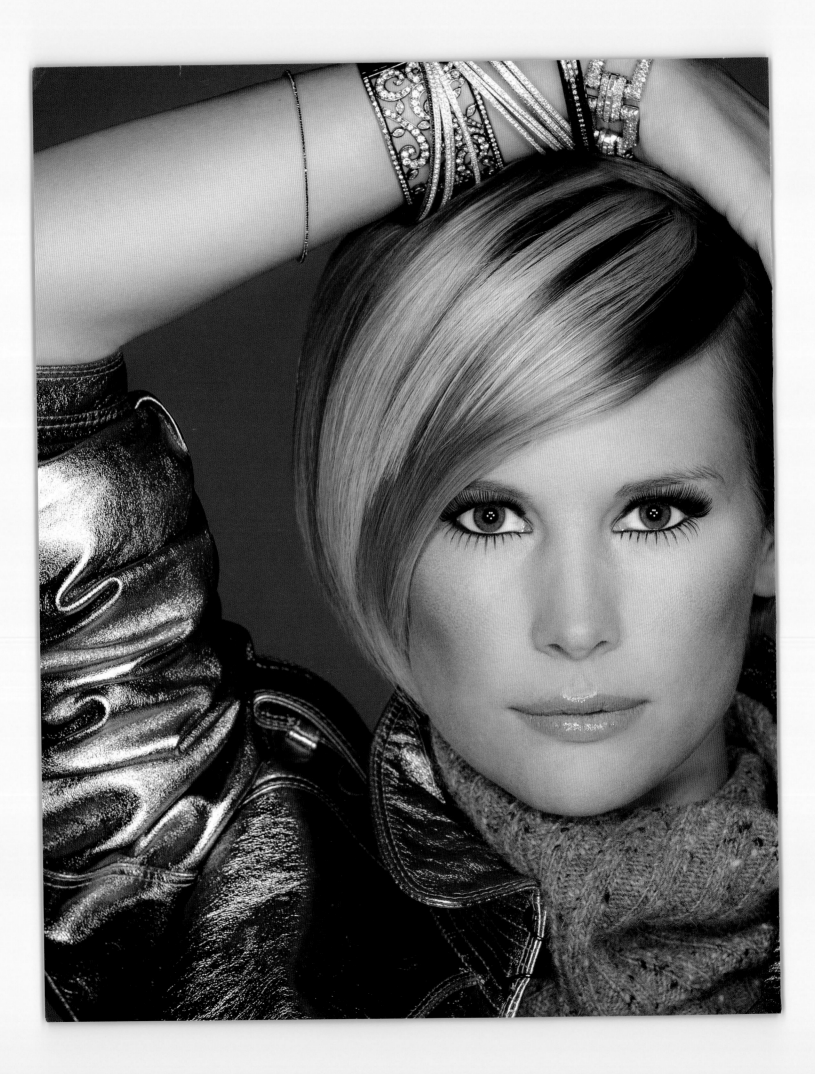

Jocelyn Goldstein (WARDROBE)

Styling in particular is something I sort of fell into, and I have had the good fortune of working with and learning from some of the best people in the industry for the past ten years. I started as an intern at Isaac Mizrahi and then moved on to an internship with the fashion director at *Vibe* magazine. It was there that I discovered that my favorite part of the job was going on shoots. So, I began working as an assistant on different editorial and ad campaigns, with my first job being on a Burberry ad campaign in Paris. I also assisted Camilla Nickerson, an editor at *Vogue* magazine, who has now moved on to *W* magazine. I continued assisting various stylists, including Andrea Lieberman, doing lots of video and print work, as well as red carpet work. Andrea continues to be a great mentor and friend. Now, I work solo on various commercial, celeb, and editorial shoots. The job itself never gets old. I still have butterflies when I work, as there is always a new challenge to face.

When Scott Barnes does makeup, it's amazing to see how expressive, yet effortless, his art can be. When we work together we are inspired by one another and work to create beautiful images. But although we can work hard to get the most amazing hair, makeup, and clothing on a person, if the beauty doesn't also come from within, it's useless.

Sometimes people have the tendency to put on everything they love all at once. But it's not necessarily about that. Fashion is so individual. It's a feeling you get when you see somebody wearing something that looks amazing, and you think, "Oh my God; that works!" Sometimes the process of dressing a model is organic, but sometimes it isn't. Ultimately, it's about trying different clothes, experimenting, and making sure the outfit makes the person look and feel beautiful. If you have confidence, you can look beautiful because you know you are beautiful.

The Power of BEAUTY

We've always been fascinated with stories of transformation. Some of the most beautiful and memorable females in history and literature are women who have gone through significant transformations. There's Eliza Doolittle, the low-class flower girl turned high-class lady in George Bernard Shaw's play, Pygmalion, who later sang her way into people's hearts in the popular musical, My Fair Lady. The Cinderella story about the ill-treated sister who becomes a princess is known by children the world over. Even Gigi, the Academy Award–winning movie musical based on the French novel of the same title, portrays an awkward teenager being groomed as a courtesan who evolves into a respectable young woman. These stories serve as wonderful morality tales about the implications of physical transformation. But in my mind, the most powerful transformation is the one found in the Bible's Book of Esther. It's the original transformation story, and I think it best depicts the power of beauty.

Esther is a young Jewish peasant girl who is ultimately selected to become the wife of the Persian king, Ahasuerus (some texts refer to him as King Xerxes). Esther uses her beauty to find favor with the king and become his queen. But the story doesn't stop there. As queen, Esther, along with her cousin Mordecai, is able to persuade the king to cancel an order for the extermination of Jews in his kingdom. Today, the Jewish festival of Purim celebrates this event.

Keep in mind that this girl was the daughter of a goat herder. Being a peasant, she was probably very dirty. She didn't wear fine clothes or jewelry, and it's doubtful she had time to comb and set her hair. So, there was definitely some grooming involved before she presented herself to the king. What's remarkable about Esther is that she could've easily viewed her success at finding favor with the king as an impossible feat. After all, the odds were certainly against her. She was a girl from humble means whose parents had died and whose faith conflicted with that of the king. Instead of giving up, though, she did what she needed to do to make herself as beautiful as possible to get the king's attention. She had an open, positive approach and saw the opportunity presented to her.

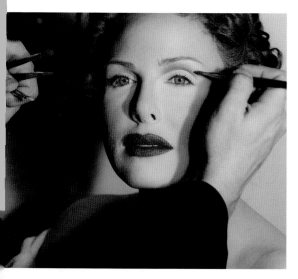

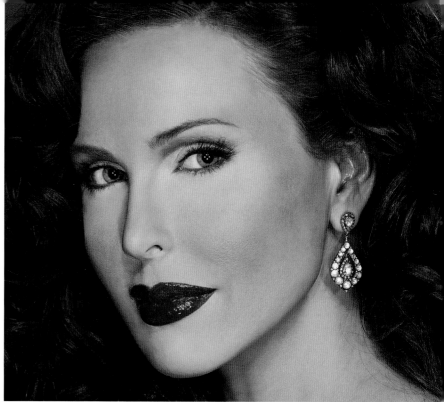

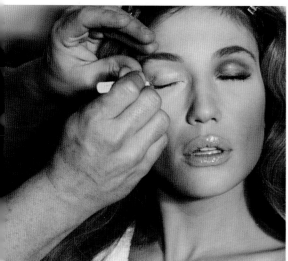

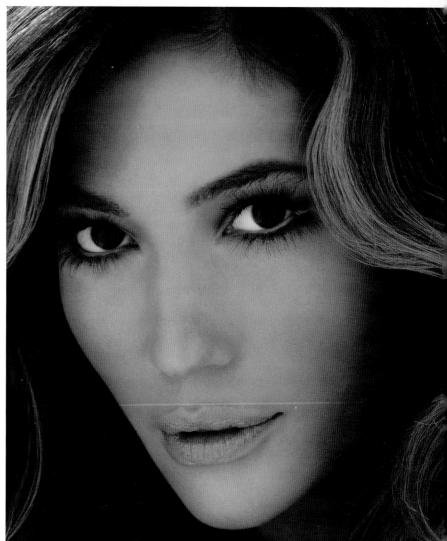

Esther made a conscious effort to be better. She actively sought the king's favor, and in so doing, she actively sought God's favor.

This story, as with the other transformation stories mentioned earlier, is not just about beauty for vanity's sake. These tales show how each woman effects change in the lives of people around them. Esther's story is the most significant in that her beauty saved the Jews from being massacred. It doesn't get more significant than saving a race of people. Her beauty led to her living a purpose-driven life. Although the king noticed Esther because of her outer beauty, it was her inner beauty, her strength of character, and her actions that influenced a positive outcome. Even in the stories of Cinderella, My Fair Lady, and Gigi, the women are more than just pretty faces. They impress others with their nobility of character. These are women of substance who because they come from more humble beginnings have a generosity of spirit, a compassion for others, and a humility that intensifies their beauty. There's grace in humility. Humility is downright sexy.

The women chosen for this book are certainly beautiful women. But as you read their stories, you will see that they are also women of substance. Something more than vanity drives them to take care of themselves. They are passionate about such things as photography, privacy, animals, and family. They are women who believe in taking care of their bodies and stimulating their minds, and they believe they have something to offer the world. Their physical transformations only help to bolster these beliefs.

One last thing: The best part about the stories of Esther, Cinderella, Eliza, and Gigi is that each of these women also finally realized she was no less important or no less worthy than the other "beautiful" people around her. Each woman gained confidence and self-worth in the process of her own transformation. It's an important point. In fact, it may even be the point: If you're doing things to make yourself feel better and look better—grooming yourself, eating well, exercising, and doing whatever it takes to become your most beautiful self—it can benefit you in extraordinary ways that stretch far beyond mere physical appearance. I think of it as empowering yourself, having a spiritual relationship with *Self.* And that's the real power of beauty.

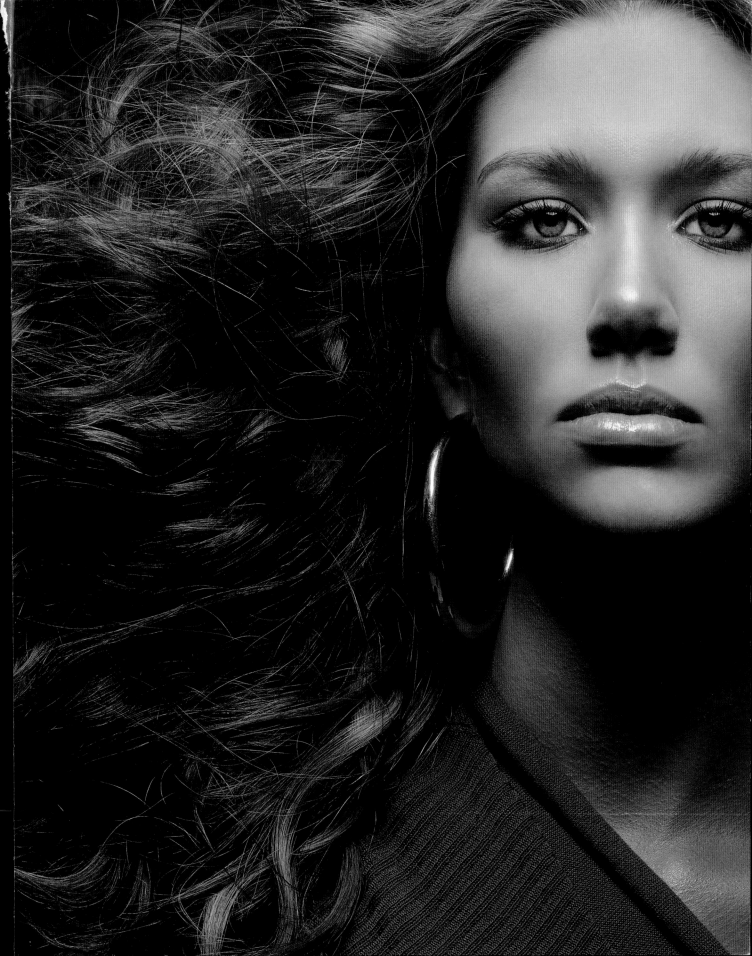

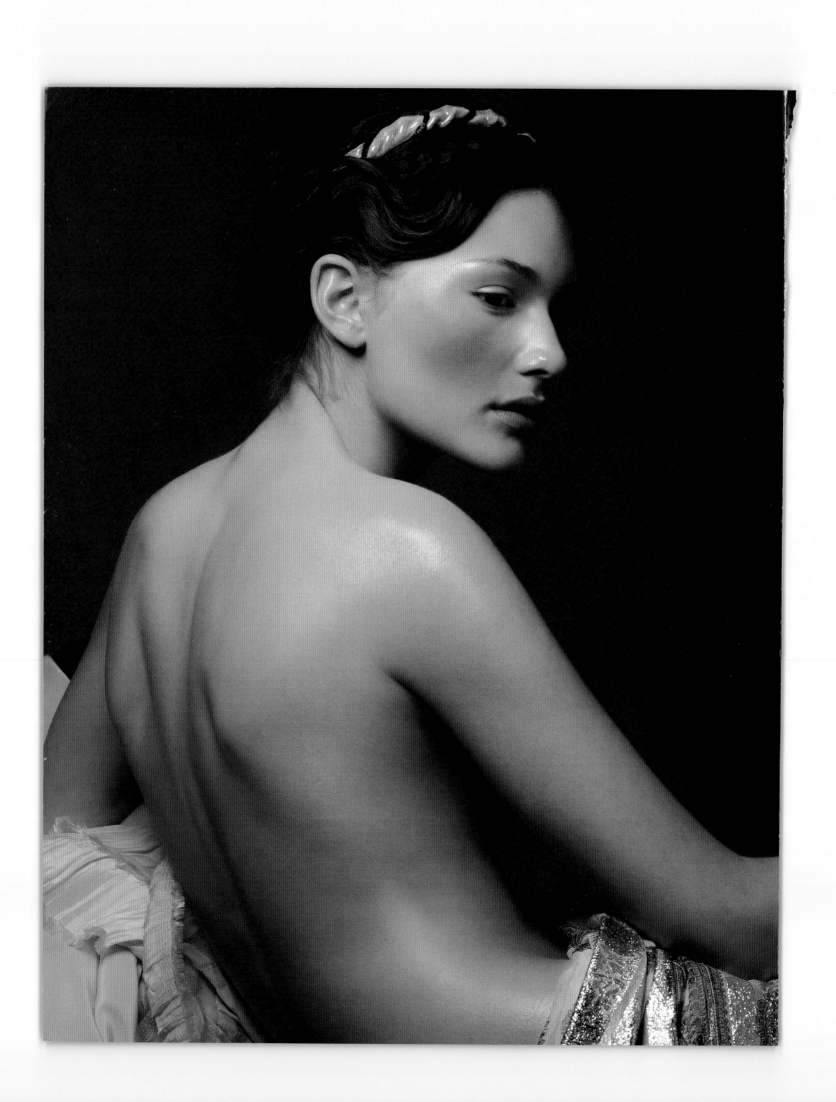

You have the power
to create your own
MASTERPIECE.
—Scott Barnes

I used both red and yellow foundations to stay as close as possible to the light and dark of her NATURAL COLORING.

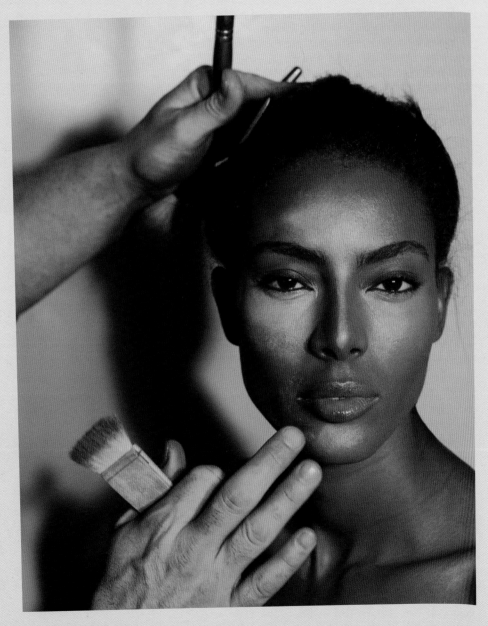

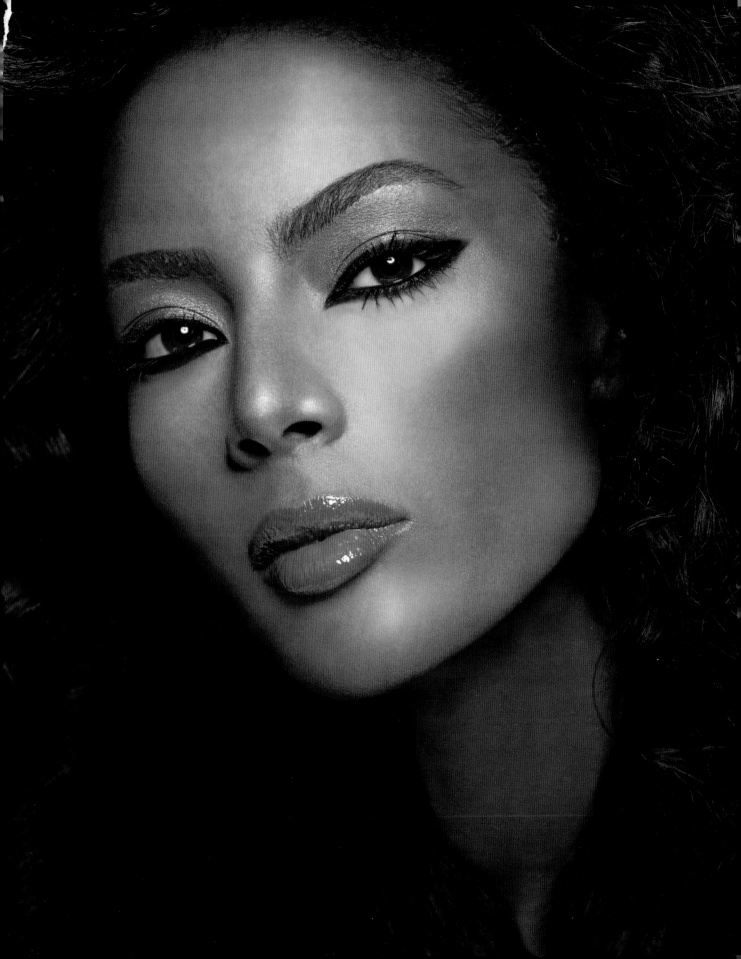

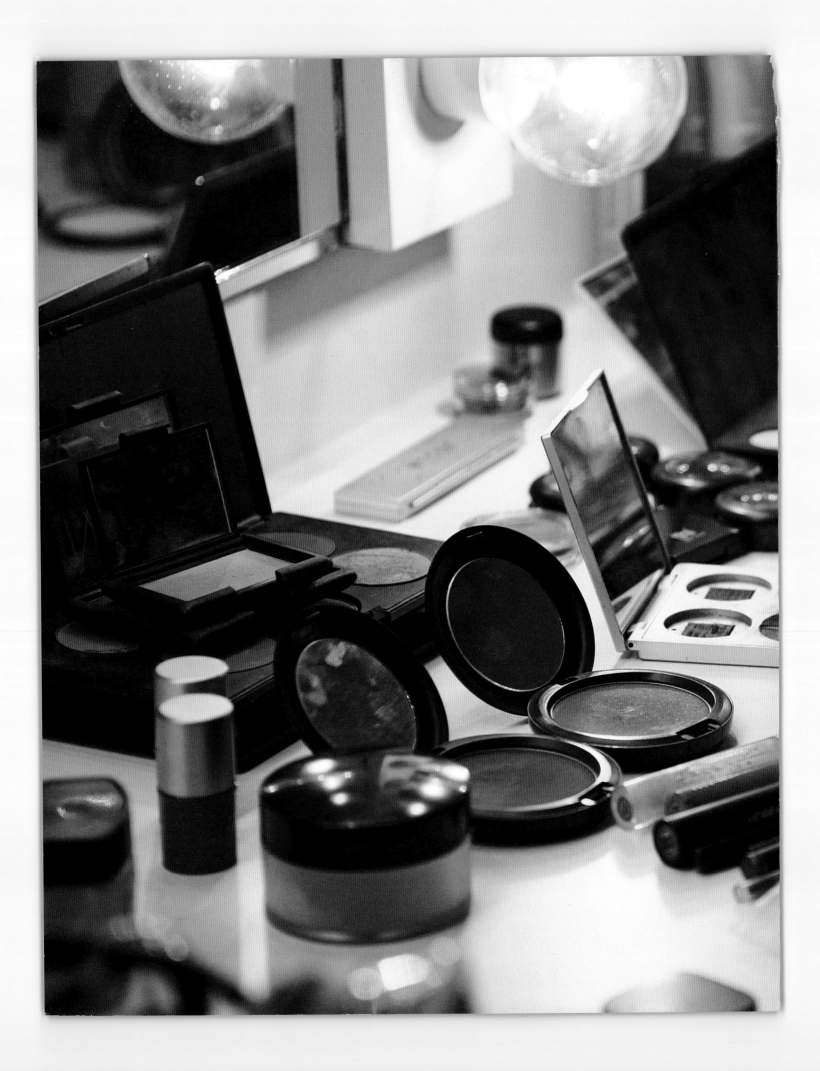

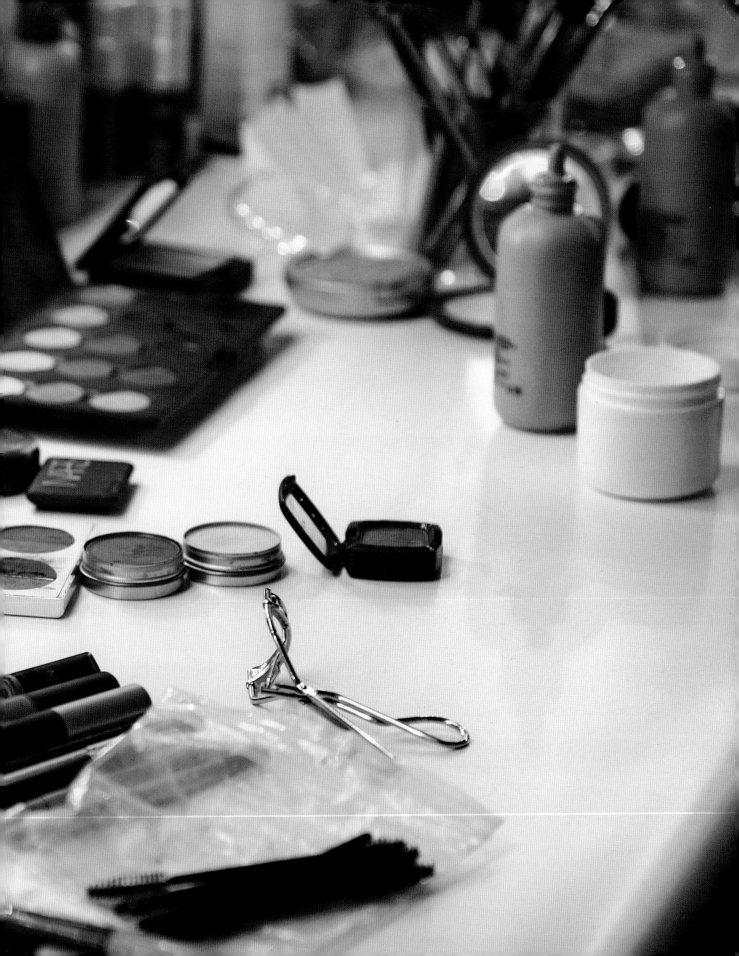

Transformations

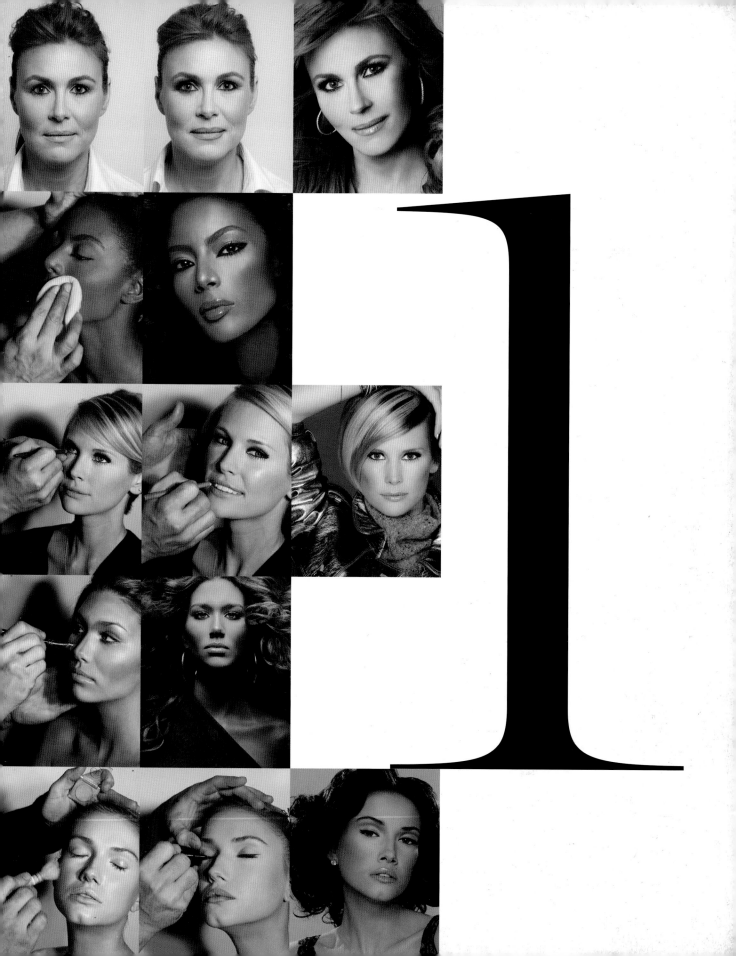

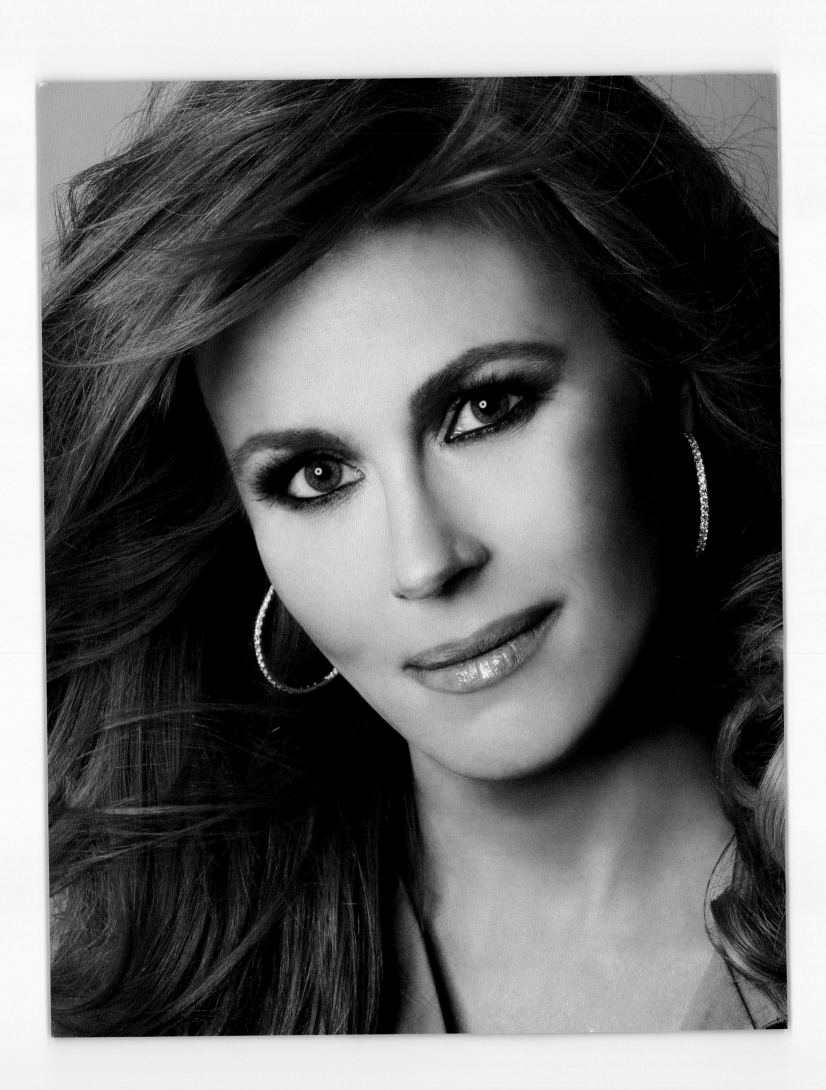

Katherine:
How to Make Glamour Work

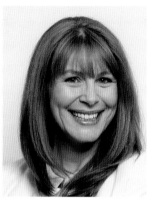

Katherine Albrecht is a well-known privacy expert. She got her doctorate in education from Harvard, she's the author of the bestselling book *Spychips*, and she hosts the syndicated radio show "Uncovering the Truth." As a freedom campaigner, she's far from the typical angry activist who doesn't know how to present herself. In fact, she's just the opposite. Katherine knows her power as a woman, and with her transformation, she's learned how she can take her femininity even further when fighting for an important cause. Now when people meet her for the first time, they're surprised by just how beautiful, how confident, and even how sexy she is. What a great way to start any conversation, even if it's with your adversary.

Scott + Katherine Talk ...

SCOTT: What is your beauty regime in the morning?

KATHERINE: It depends on whether I'm going out into the world or whether I'm working in my home office. Typically, even if I'm working from home, I will wash my face with a washcloth and water. Pretty straightforward, nothing fancy. I have really dry skin, especially in the wintertime, so my biggest problem is not to remove oil; it's what's keeping my skin moisturized.

SCOTT: Right, water's actually better for your skin than soap, because water leaves some of your natural oils behind. It's like leaving natural oils in your hair.

KATHERINE: Yes, exactly. And when I do use a cleanser, usually when I need to remove a lot of makeup, I try to use really rich, creamy cleansers. Then I follow that up with a moisturizer. For makeup, I typically put on just a little bit of foundation, because I kind of need it. My skin's a little blotchy and freckly,

(continued on page 35)

Creating Katherine's Look

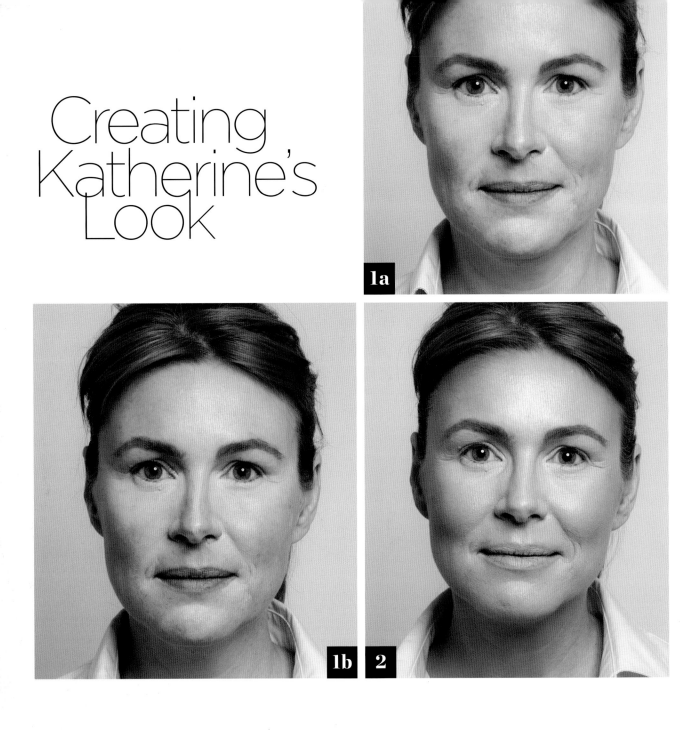

1a

1b 2

Tip To find the apples of your cheeks...simply smile.

Katherine told me the thing she struggled with most was her eyes. She knew they were small, but she felt that eye makeup made them look even smaller. Her eyes are a great color—a pale gray-blue-green—so I set out to show her how she could get more wow power with them.

....

1 Contouring, highlighting, and foundation

Katherine has a healthy complexion with a lot of red undertones. I wanted to alleviate some of the redness in her skin by using a pinky-beige color for her foundation and give her a more unified tone overall. **(a)** Using light strokes with a goat hair brush, I applied a cream contouring (dark) foundation: ● Underneath the jaw line ● Underneath the cheekbones ● On the sides of the nose ● At the temples ● Under the tip of the nose (to give the illusion of shortening the nose) **(b)** Using a goat hair concealer brush, I applied a cream highlighting (light) concealer: ● On top of the cheekbones ● In the center of the forehead ● Under the eyes ● Underneath the eyebrows ● On the bridge of the nose ● At the center of the chin **(c)** Using a third goat hair brush, I applied a cream pinky-beige foundation on top of the contouring and highlighting and blended by moving the brush in a circular motion for a smooth, seamless transition.

2 Cheeks

I used a coral blush that matched her natural lip tone and applied the blush on the apples of her cheeks, moving the blush brush in small circles.

Tip Katherine has red hair. In addition to matching her natural lip tone, coral is also good on a redhead because it has a lot of yellow in it which complements red hair; however, it still has enough pink in it so that the effect isn't muddy-looking.

(continued from page 33)

so I put on just a little bit of a very light, light foundation. I usually follow that with a little lipstick, a dash of eye shadow, a little mascara, and I'm good to go.

SCOTT: How would you define "beautiful"?
KATHERINE: I think "beautiful" is silky, glowing hair glowing skin, healthy skin, and overall good health. If you don't feel healthy, it shows, even with all the makeup in the world. There's a difference in your posture and everything else about you when you feel good. There's an element of sexy in beauty, too. It's that feminine thing that so many of us forget to project as we become busy with other things, especially those of us who have been married a long time. But I think if you really want to have the va-voom kind of beauty, there's an element of sexy that you need to put back into your beauty regimen.

SCOTT: Do you think a person can be smart and sexy?
KATHERINE: Absolutely, I think they totally go hand in hand. For the past ten years my job as an activist has been to intimidate men specifically. Ninety percent of the people I deal with

(continued on page 37)

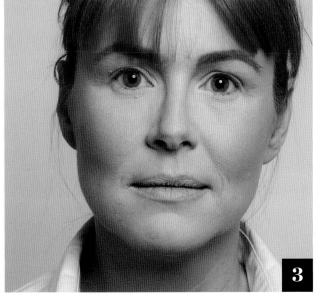

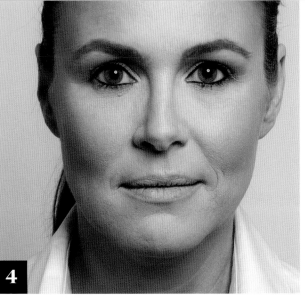

3 **4**

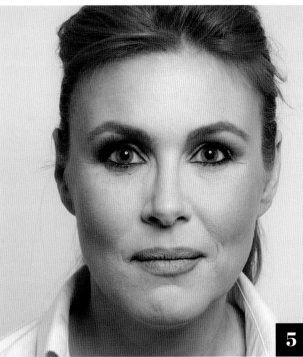

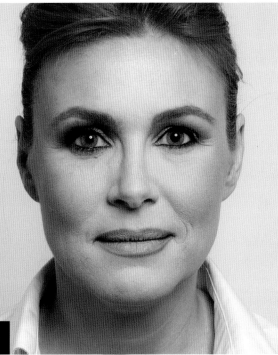

5 **6**

Tip For eyelashes that stay curled, hold down the eyelash curler for a count of 20 and then apply mascara immediately.

Tip For redheads, lining the eyelid with a brown pencil helps bring out the eyes, while still being a softer, more natural look than lining with a black pencil.

(continued from page 35)

3 Eyebrows

Katherine's eyebrows were in pretty good shape, so I trimmed them only minimally to clean them up. I also filled them in with a mustard-colored eye shadow using an angled brow brush. Katherine has brown eyebrows, so I put yellow shadow on them to bring out more red in her eyebrows to compliment her red hair since the combination of brown and yellow makes red!

4 Eyes

Most redheads have light eyes, and Katherine is no exception. Her eyes are a beautiful pale gray-blue-green, which deserve to be highlighted. **(a)** For the eye shadow base, I selected a color two shades darker than her hair—a reddish brown color—and brushed it over the whole eye. **(b)** Then with a different eye shadow brush, I applied a darker chocolate brown shadow into the crease, under the eye, on the top of the lid by the lash line. **(c)** I then lined the inside rim of her eye with a chocolate brown pencil. Note: Katherine could easily switch out this brown liner for black liner to create a more dramatic look for special events. **(d)** Finally, I curled her eyelashes and applied lots of black mascara, which provides more drama than brown mascara. The end result is a much fuller, thicker, bolder eye that doesn't look too harsh or heavily made up since I used brown-toned eye shadow and liner instead of Katherine's typical black eyeliner look.

5 Lips

Redheads have a tendency to go red-brown with their lipstick, which I think is a mistake. The darker color draws focus away from the eyes and clashes with the hair. It's usually better to go with a lighter-colored lipstick instead of a darker color to avoid the lip color overpowering the rest of your lighter features, particularly your eyes. **(a)** I lined Katherine's lips with a pale auburn liner to draw her hair color back into her face. **(b)** I then applied a pale coral gloss since I didn't want to make the whole lip auburn.

6 Setting the look

I finished off with a nice dusting of translucent powder so as not to change the color of the foundation and the blush. Using a large powder brush, I lightly swept the powder all over her face and neck for an even finish.

are men, and they're some of the most powerful corporate executives in the world. I think a smart and powerful woman can be intimidating to men, but I think femininity in general— being a powerful, sexy woman—can be even more intimidating.

SCOTT: Do you think it's important to be beautiful in your line of work?
KATHERINE: I think a woman can be extremely smart and competent, but when she adds that extra layer of "beauty," it's as if people are able to see her competence more quickly.

REACTIONS...

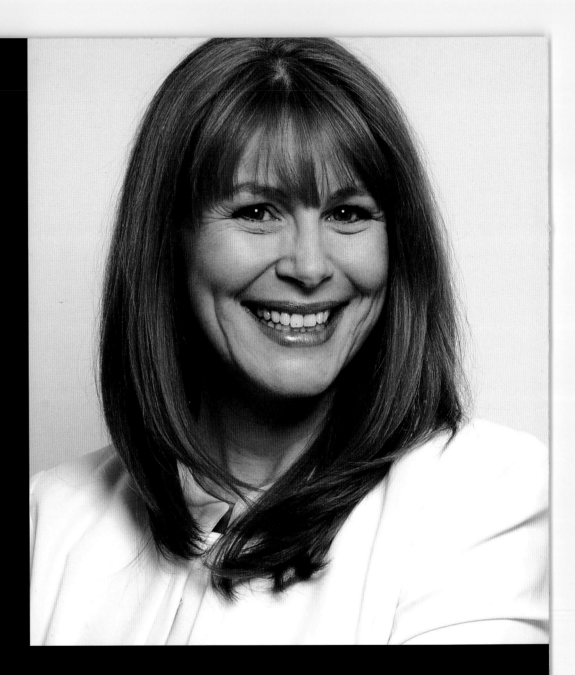

Katherine's Reaction to Her Transformation

"I've learned that there's a little bit of an extra edge that comes from being a beautiful, strong, powerful woman, particularly when you're having an open debate with men. Breaking down the stereotype of the mean, ugly, negative, angry female activist is a part of my power. I love the fact that Scott has helped me to break through that activist stereotype even more with a new look, especially since I believe that looking and feeling my best helps attract more people to the cause. Who wants to follow an angry, ugly person? People would much rather follow somebody who's positive and who feels really good about herself."

"Before, I was the confident, professional businesswoman, but now I also have the ability to be over-the-top glamorous, if I choose. And people treat you very differently when you possess both qualities. In fact, just the other day, I had to travel to Los Angeles for a meeting, and I had literally forgotten to pack my makeup in

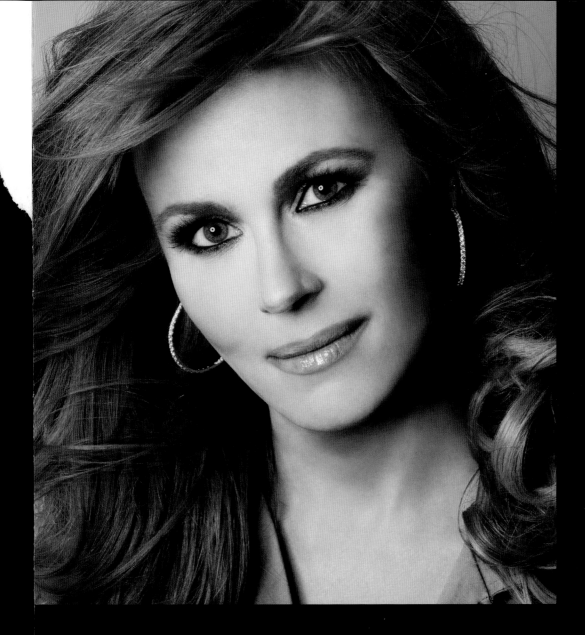

my suitcase, so I had nothing to put on except pale pink lipstick. Here I was with my glasses on and my pale pink lipstick and my hair pulled back in a ponytail, and it was so funny because the guy I met told me how great my photo was on my website. But his subtext was…'and you're not really that pretty in person.' So, I went out during our lunch break, bought $100 worth of makeup, sat in my car, and did the whole Scott Barnes makeover and then went back to the meeting. That same guy

and everybody else around him treated me like I was a different person. You can tell, it's like night and day… a different level of appreciation and admiration that people treat you with when you do the whole Scott Barnes makeup thing. They treat you like you're more competent, like you are more 'deserving' of their respect. I didn't feel disrespected before, but there's definitely a feeling that you're one of the people in charge of the situation, instead of one of the people in the background."

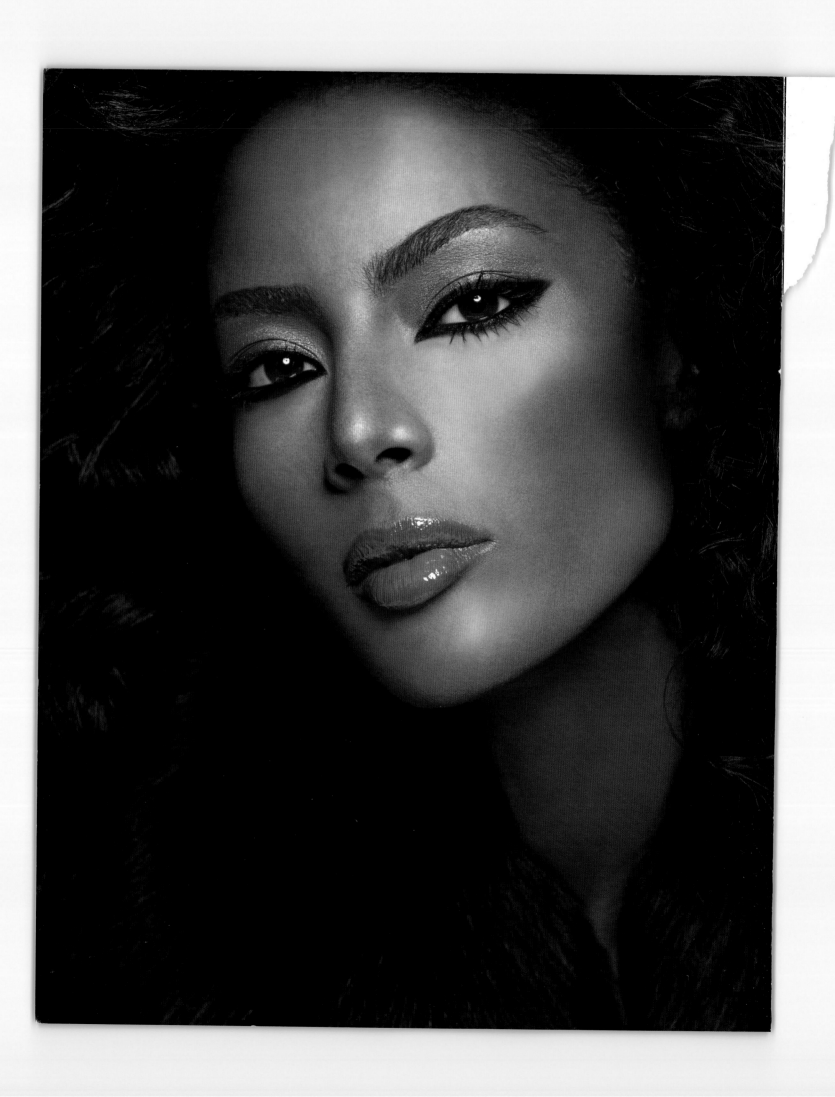

Gate:
Combining Earth Tones for a Monochromatic Look

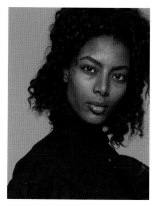

There's a long-standing debate about whether Egypt was settled by Africans or Europeans. Gate, a model, is Ethiopian. She made a point of telling me this when I remarked that her bone structure and features reminded me of the ancient Egyptians. She went on to explain that Ethiopia is "mixed" and consists of people from many different parts of the world—Africa, India, Egypt, Italy, Yemen, and Israel—and that her parents are black Ethiopians. I did a bit of research and discovered that Ethiopians—and Somalis in particular—are said to most closely resemble the ancient Egyptians and Nubians. Some sociologists believe, in fact, that Egyptians are actually descendents of Ethiopians who migrated into Egypt. That fits with my perception of Gate as an Egyptian princess. Perhaps it has more to do with the regal way she carries herself. Or maybe it's because her actions are also stately. Her husband, who is the chef for the five-star restaurant, Aquavit, introduced Gate to UNICEF. Now, in addition to modeling, she works with UNICEF on Africa–U.S. relations. Gate is a beautiful woman with an admirable nobility of character, and she deserves a look that's equally distinguished.

SCOTT: What is your typical diet?

GATE: I'm not really picky, but I know what I like. I love food, but I don't really eat junk food. I'm married to a chef, so I eat very healthy food everyday. He cooks, and teaches me things. So even when he's not home, I make myself a nice chicken dish or fish dish or a salad. I like lamb...soft meat...not cow meat. I like to eat, so I exercise almost every day.

SCOTT: What kind of exercise do you do?

GATE: I take a West African dance class. I also do yoga, play basketball, and go biking. I also walk a lot every day, which is also a good workout.

SCOTT: Do you wear a lot of makeup usually?

GATE: No, I wear no makeup when I'm not working. I just want my skin fresh. I used to wear a lot of makeup, but my skin was getting irritated by using a lot of different products. So, when I'm not working, I just wear mascara and lip gloss, so I can let my skin rest from having to wear makeup.

(continued on page 43)

Creating Gate's Look

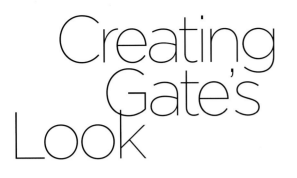

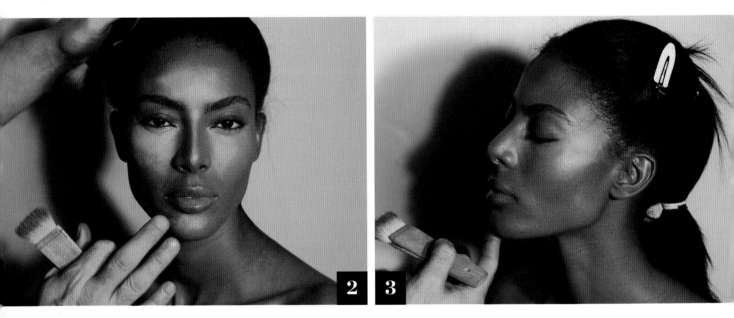

Tip Women with dark skin should have two or three foundations that they can blend on the face to create a more natural-looking foundation with greater dimension. Dark skin is never one color; usually it has two or three tones. So, when applying foundation you want to try to mimic the natural coloring of these different tones. Otherwise, you risk flattening out the face and making it either too light or too dark overall using only one color.

Gate's Reaction to Her Transformation

"I was like...wow! I looked and felt totally different! Scott didn't put a lot of makeup on my face, but he knew about my coloring and just what I needed. Many makeup artists use so much more makeup."

"I've tried all kinds of makeup before. I've been in the modeling industry for five years, and I haven't found one foundation that I really love. Because of my dark skin, I need yellows and reds. And the way he applied my foundation was perfect for my skin. And the concealer he used looks amazing. It evens out my skin and goes on so easily."

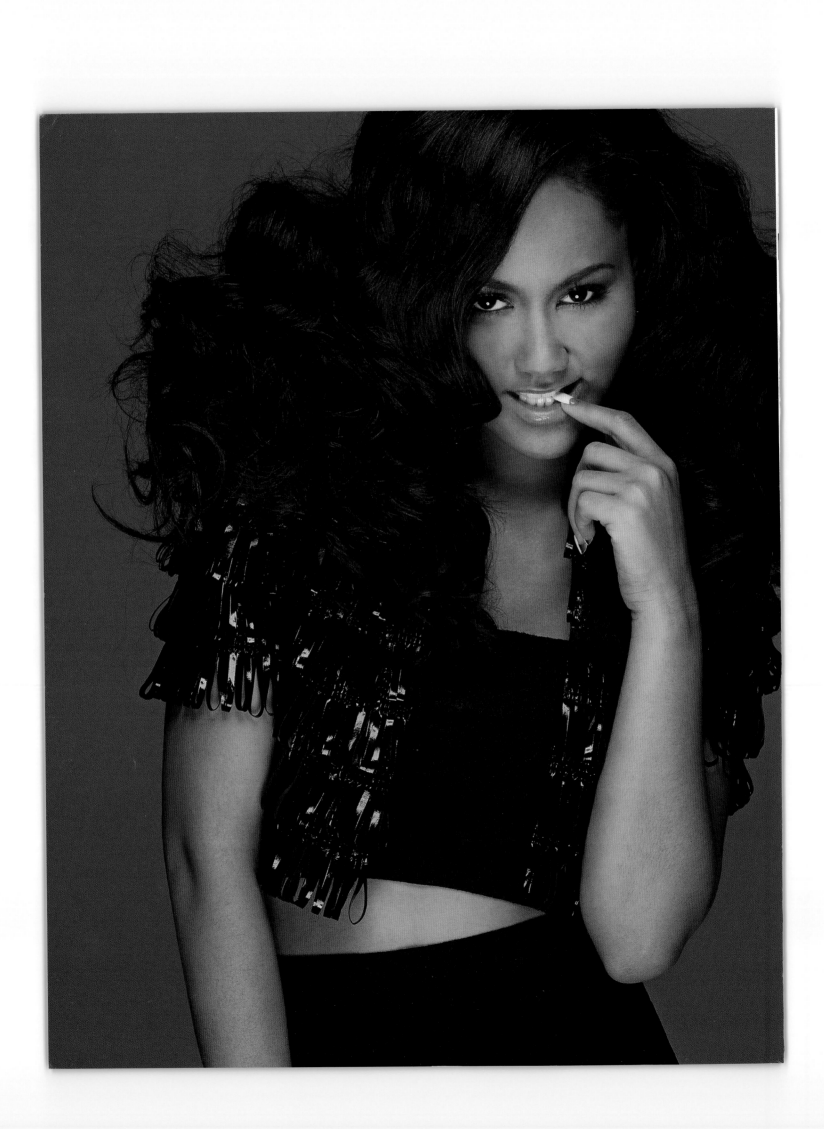

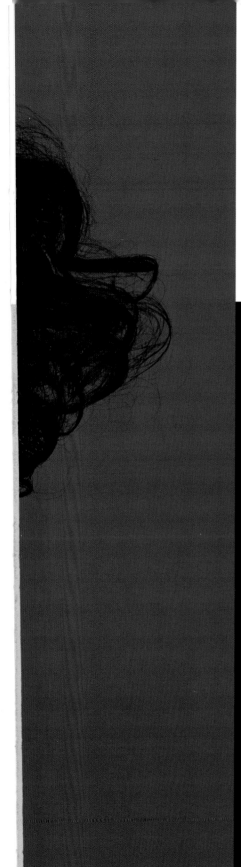

Kat DeLuna ★

Since she's such an
AUTHENTIC TALENT,
I wanted to see
Kat with a look that
was more unique,
something she
could really own.

Scott on Kat

Kat describes herself as an up-and-coming artist, and I predict it won't be long before the rest of the world catches on to her talent. She's the real thing—not just another marketing package—with all the right stuff to become a huge success. Being classically trained in opera, Kat can sing like a bird. Or she can do down-and-dirty pop. This girl's got range, with a voice that'll knock your socks off. And have you seen her dance?! To watch her move, you'd never guess she was never formally trained.

Since she's such an authentic talent, I wanted to see Kat with a look that was more unique, something she could really own. Kat is from the Dominican Republic, so I encouraged her to drop the blonde look and go back to her natural coloring. Her Latin roots are very important to her, so she liked the idea of going with a style that supports who she is and what she believes in. Her fan base keeps growing, so it seems they've embraced the new Kat. There's a lot that's special about this bilingual singer-songwriter, and I look forward to watching her wind ...all the way to the top.

REACTIONS...

(continued from page 57)

SCOTT: Do you have any kind of philosophy when it comes to beauty?

LOUISA: Do everything in moderation—even moderation. I think life is meant to be enjoyed. There's always so much "do this, don't do that" and "eat this, don't eat that." I think it should be about maintaining a well-balanced approach. When people who know me see me drinking coffee, they think "that's a little hypocritical" because I'm always talking about nutrition. But I'm pretty healthy overall, so my one espresso in the morning isn't going to shut me down. I can go without the coffee, but it makes me happy, so I feel it's okay to allow myself such things as long as I do it in moderation.

SCOTT: Do you have any plans once you're no longer modeling?

LOUISA: On the weekends, I'm in nutrition school. I'm already working toward becoming a holistic health counselor. I've got a website and a few clients rolling in already! That's my new focus lately, which in addition to everything else is keeping me super busy.

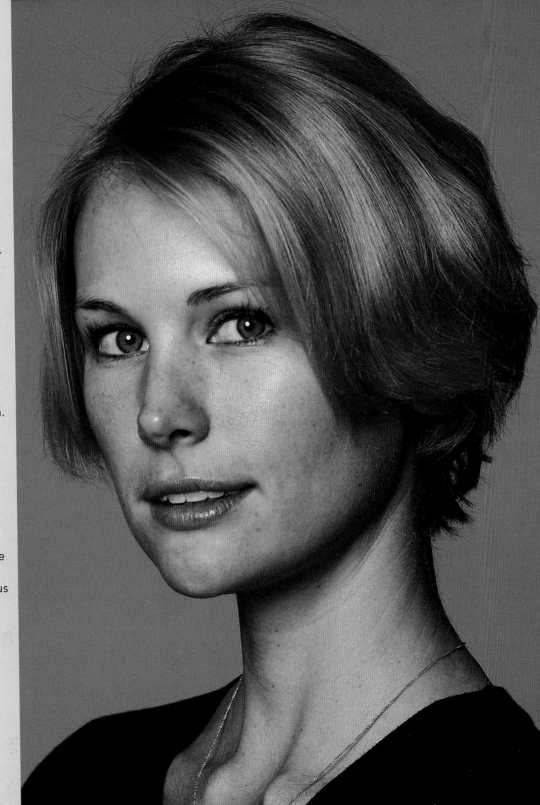

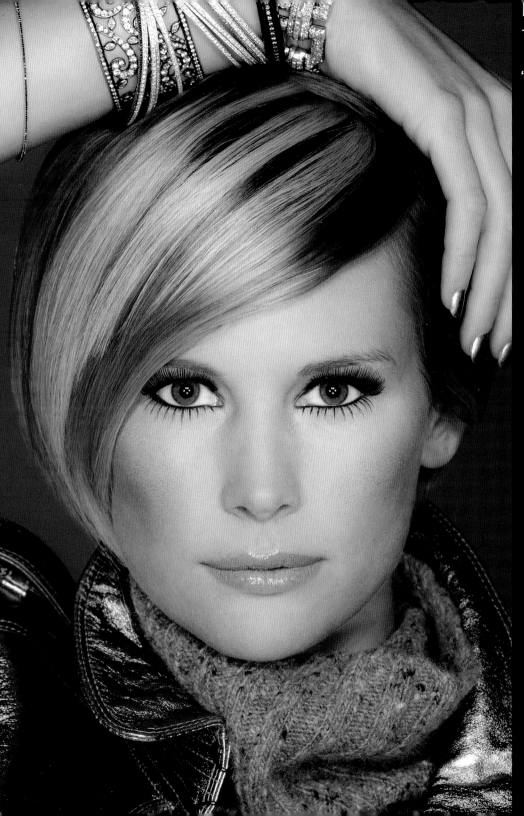

Louisa's Reaction to Her Transformation

"I look great! Compared to other makeup artists Scott took a 'less is more' approach. Everything looks fairly natural but has such impact. The whole process was super simple. For starters, Scott didn't cake on the foundation or powder like most makeup artists do. And he totally worked my eyes. He explained to me that my eyes are a little deep-set, so some extra liner and some lashes will go a long way to make them pop. And it's so true. I definitely work the liner more now. I don't wear a lot of makeup unless I'm going out, but when I do, I now know I can focus on the eyes and lashes."

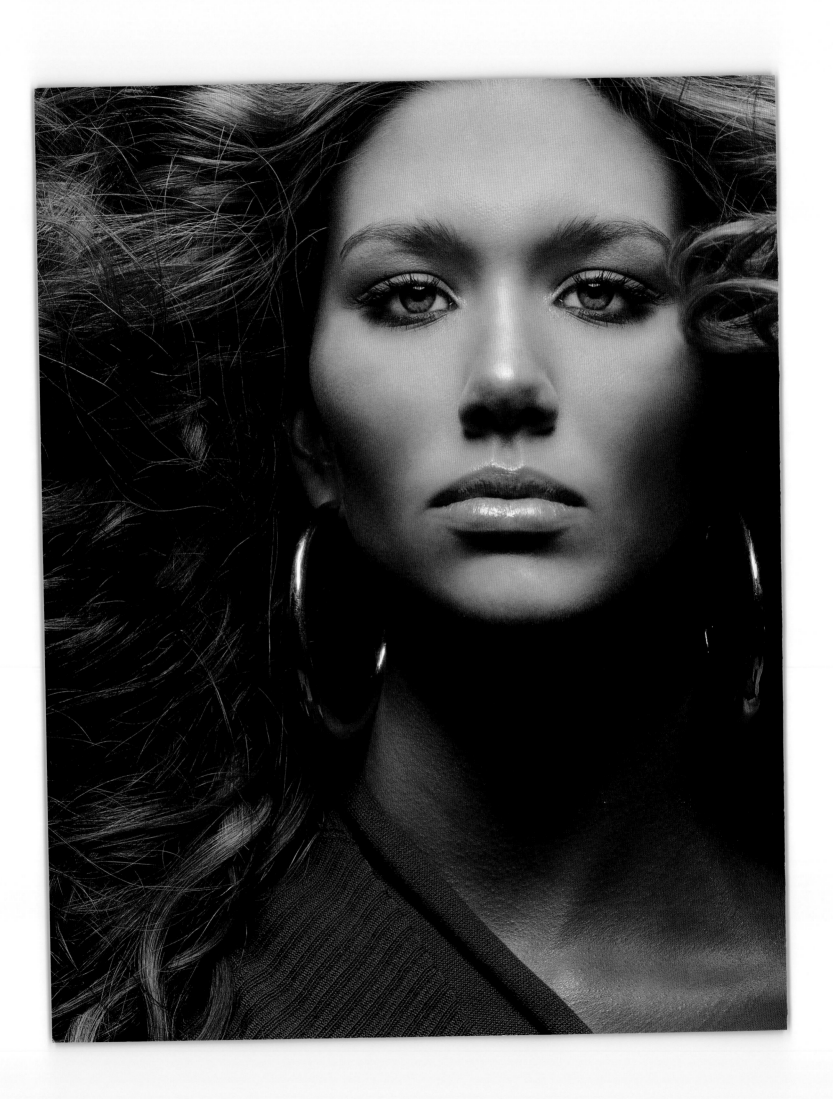

Jessica:
Creating a Believable Faux Tan for Face and Body

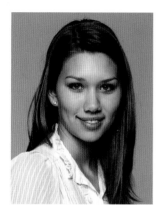

Jessica's dream is to become a freelance artist. As a studio art major at New York University, Jessica balances her time between a full course load at NYU and a part-time modeling career. At nineteen years old, she comes across as a highly disciplined, extremely pragmatic individual. She's already focusing on landing an internship, stating that "as fun as it would be to be an artist showing my work in galleries, it's kind of dicey to try to make a living doing only that." So, she's decided to explore the art direction and media side of the art world as her backup plan.

Jessica has terrifically blue eyes, but her skin tone is more golden than that of a typical Caucasian, so I asked about her nationality. She told me she was a mix between Irish, Scottish, German, and a bit of Cherokee Indian and that she gets "really dark in the summer." Perfect. I could easily picture her on a beach somewhere in the Caribbean. But I wanted to show her how she could get that same deep tan without spending so much time in the sun, damaging her skin. Bronze goddess, here we come.

SCOTT: What do you think are your best features?
JESSICA: I always thought my eyes were probably my best feature—and my hair.

SCOTT: You have lots of hair.
JESSICA: I know, and I never, ever brush it, which is probably not good, but I have a sensitive scalp; besides, I kind of like the messier look, it's more me. I'm a natural, very low-key girl when it comes to styling. If I'm going out, I'll blow out my hair and then throw on some product to give it some volume, scrunch, and go. Or I'll just throw my hair up in a bun. I'm also low-key with my makeup. If I do wear makeup, it's very light. I usually wear very subtle eye shadow, if I wear any at all, like a light brown or something in an earth tone. I'll also throw on mascara, which is pretty much my staple—and lip gloss.

(continued on page 63)

Creating, Jessica's Look

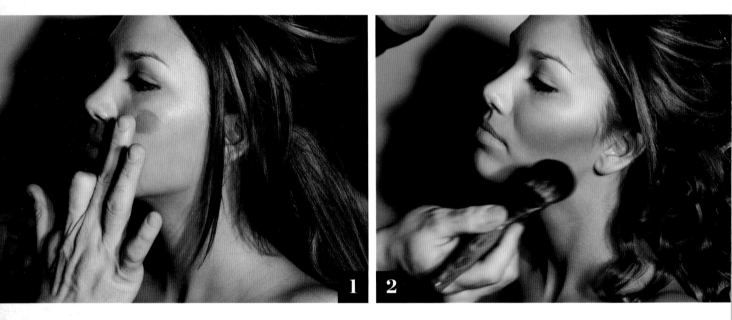

Tip Remember to blend until all the colors are married together, for a smooth finish with no separation of colors.

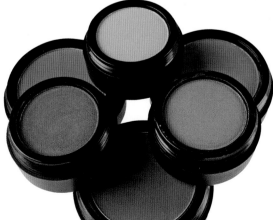

Jessica seemed pleased when she talked about getting really tan in the summer. I don't blame her—everybody feels better with a bit of color. Fortunately for her, she has some Cherokee in her, so her skin tans easily without burning. Still, we all know how damaging those ultra violet rays can be and how quickly skin ages when overexposed to the sun. So, it was important to show Jessica how she could create a faux tan and feel just as beautiful as if it were the real thing.

1 Contouring, highlighting, and foundation

For Jessica, it was about creating a unilateral tan all over her body that required minimal contouring and highlighting. **(a)** I started with Jessica's body and applied Body Bling all over to fake a tan. The trick with applying Body Bling, as with applying any kind of makeup, is—you guessed it—blending thoroughly! Keep smoothing it into your skin so that it mixes with your natural oils and so that you don't end up with darker patches anywhere. **(b)** Once her body was sufficiently bronzed, I moved on to her face. Jessica felt her nose was "too wide," so I showed her how to slim it with contouring. Using a goat hair brush, I applied contouring (dark) foundation: ● On both sides of Jessica's nose **(c)** I used bronze cream foundation that matched the bronze of her body and applied it with a goat hair brush all over her face, moving the large brush in a circular motion. **(d)** Using a smaller highlighter brush, I dusted Shimmer Highlight: ● On top of the cheekbones ● On the forehead

2 Cheeks

I applied a reddish-tan cream blush to the apples of her cheeks, blending in small circles. I chose that color to mimic a sun-kissed look.

(continued from page 61)

SCOTT: Is there anything you don't like about yourself?
JESSICA: My nose has always been something that I look at in the mirror and think, "Oh, I wish it were different." It just seems a little wide. But I would never consider surgery. So, I'm learning to embrace it. And then there are my shoulders. They're really bony. I've done everything I can to work on that in the gym, and nothing seems to work.

SCOTT: How often do you get to the gym?
JESSICA: I try to go to the gym as much as possible. With my schedule, that works out to about three or four times a week. I'll spend thirty to forty-five minutes in the cardio room on the elliptical machine or the stationary bike. Then I'll lift some weights to work on my arms.

SCOTT: How about your skincare routine? Do you do anything on a regular basis?
JESSICA: I take a shower pretty much every night. That's when I'll wash my face and then follow that up with moisturizer. I try to keep my face and my body well moisturized. I like to use cocoa butter lotion because it's really good for your skin. I also exfoliate once a week.

(continued on page 65)

Even though the colors
I used are very similar to
one another, they still ideally
require **SEPARATE BRUSHES**
for application.

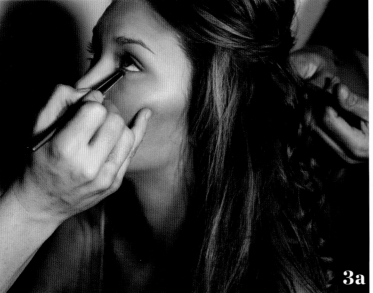

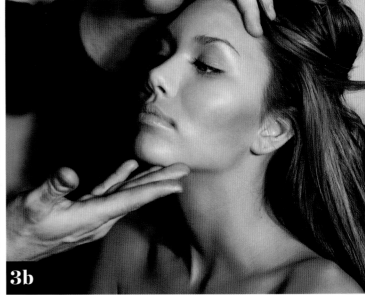

3a 3b

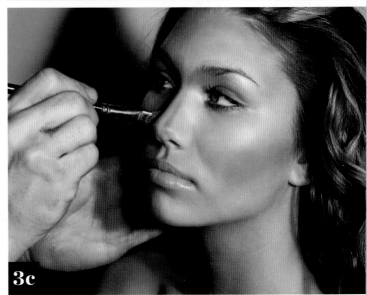

3c

(continued from page 63)

SCOTT: Sounds like you're doing all the right things. How about eating habits?

JESSICA: I was raised on a vegetarian diet. I'll eat red meat every once in a while, but I've always stayed away from chicken. But I love fish. My mom used to cook white fish or tuna or swordfish. But since I've been living at NYU, I eat dorm food.

SCOTT: How's that going?

JESSICA: Let's just say I miss my mom's cooking.

3 Eyes

The goal was to keep the look as natural as possible, so I avoided applying a lot of color and lining to Jessica's eyes. Even though the colors I used are very similar to one another, they still ideally require separate brushes for application. If you don't have separate brushes, just be sure to wipe the excess color off your brush before moving on to the next color. **(a)** I lined the lower rim of her eyes with a golden-peachy eye shadow to bring out the blue in Jessica's eyes. **(b)** I applied copper eye shadow all over her upper eyelids—from brow to lash, inside to outside corner. **(c)** I lined the lower eyelids with auburn eyeliner pencil. I used a color with a reddish tint that would appear as if she had no makeup on but would still help to accentuate her blue eyes.

4 Lips

I completed the look by adding sheer lip gloss. Jessica already had nice full lips, so no lip liner was necessary for this all-natural look.

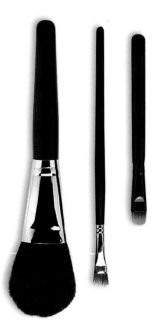

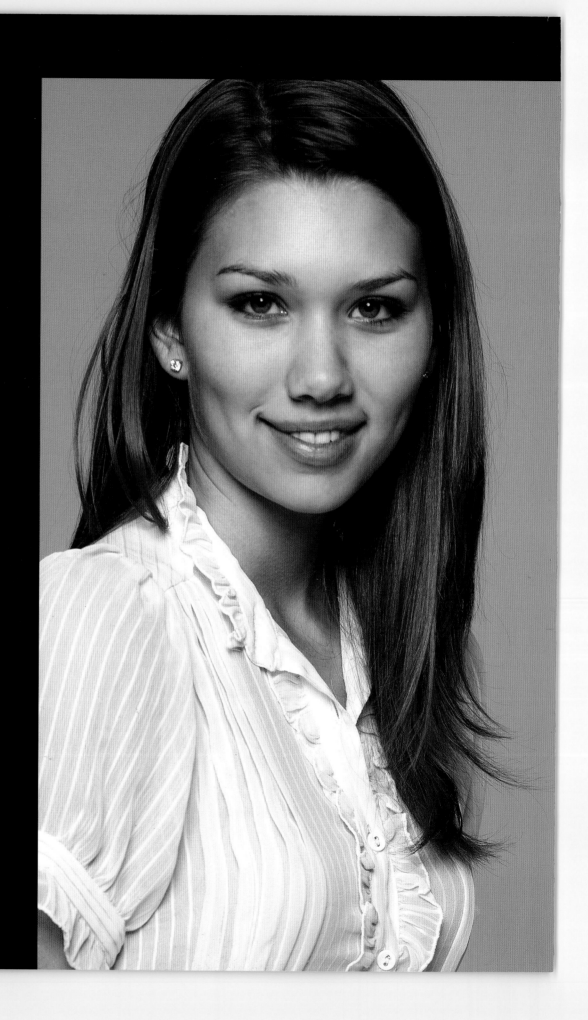

REACTIONS...

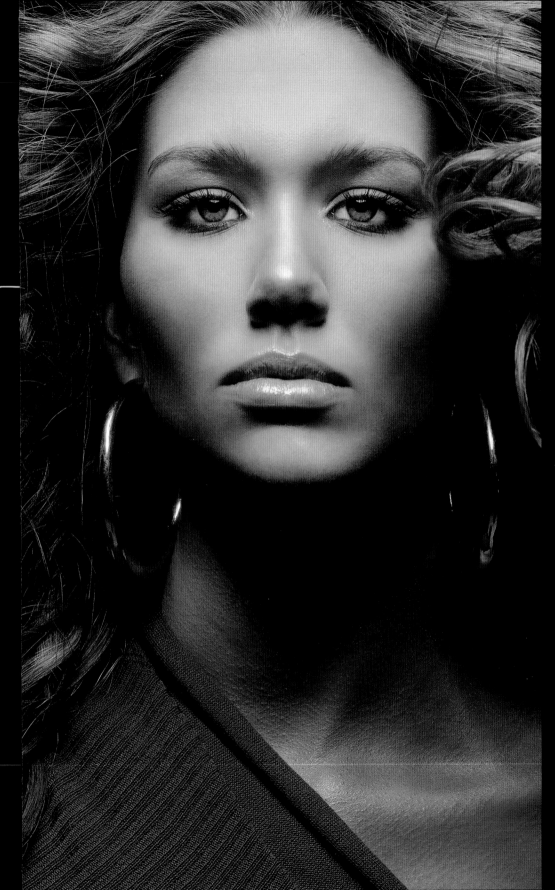

Jessica's Reaction to Her Transformation

"I look like I just came off the beach!"

"It's crazy, because I've never seen myself look quite like this with makeup. It's really amazing what can be done with makeup to change the way your whole face and body look. It's like plastic surgery without the surgery. I'm so impressed. And it's good to finally learn how to apply bronzer. Scott showed me that it's all about blending and making everything even. It's nice to know that I can achieve this look without spending a lot of time in the sun."

"I really do feel beautiful—like a bronze goddess. And it's only makeup! That's just crazy."

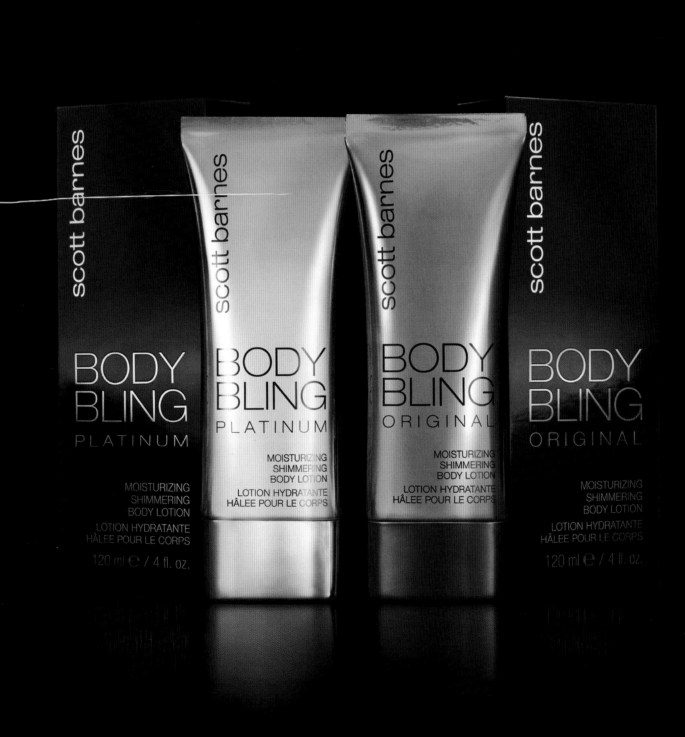

Scott Barnes on Self-Tanning

There are several faux tanning techniques, including self-tanners or bronzers. I created Body Bling™ as an alternative to the sun for immediate results. Self-tanners take a few hours to develop, and sometime have an unpleasant odor. Whether using self-tanners or bronzers, alone or in combination, the results are stunning and saves your skin. Here are some tips to glow like a pro.

FACE

The biggest no-no when applying self-tanner to the face is putting too much lotion underneath your eyes, in the creases of your nose or mouth, or anyplace where, if you go darker, it will age you, such as in the creases of your skin. You want to try to create a halo around the face with the tanning solution, while keeping those areas in the center of your face a little lighter.

BODY

It's really important to cover your nails and palms with rubber gloves. Roll the gloves down below your wrist in such a way that you keep your palms covered but most of the top of your hand is exposed. Rub the solution all over your body, and when you're finished, take the gloves off and rub the remaining lotion toward the ends of your fingers. This keeps the color minimal on your hands so that you avoid creating darker "monkey knuckles."

Also remember to cover your toenails (Scotch tape or Band-Aids work well). This ensures that you don't get yellow toenails or cuticles.

There's always the challenge of reaching your back. The easiest solution is to invite a friend over to help you. Have your own little tanning party: a "you tan my back, I'll tan yours" kind of thing. You can also try using a tanning spray, which sometimes helps you reach the center of your back a little more easily.

If you do make a mistake, such as making your elbows or your knees too dark, don't panic. Use Veet or some such hair removal product, which removes tanning color like it removes hair, only faster. Apply it for 30 seconds or less and then wipe away.

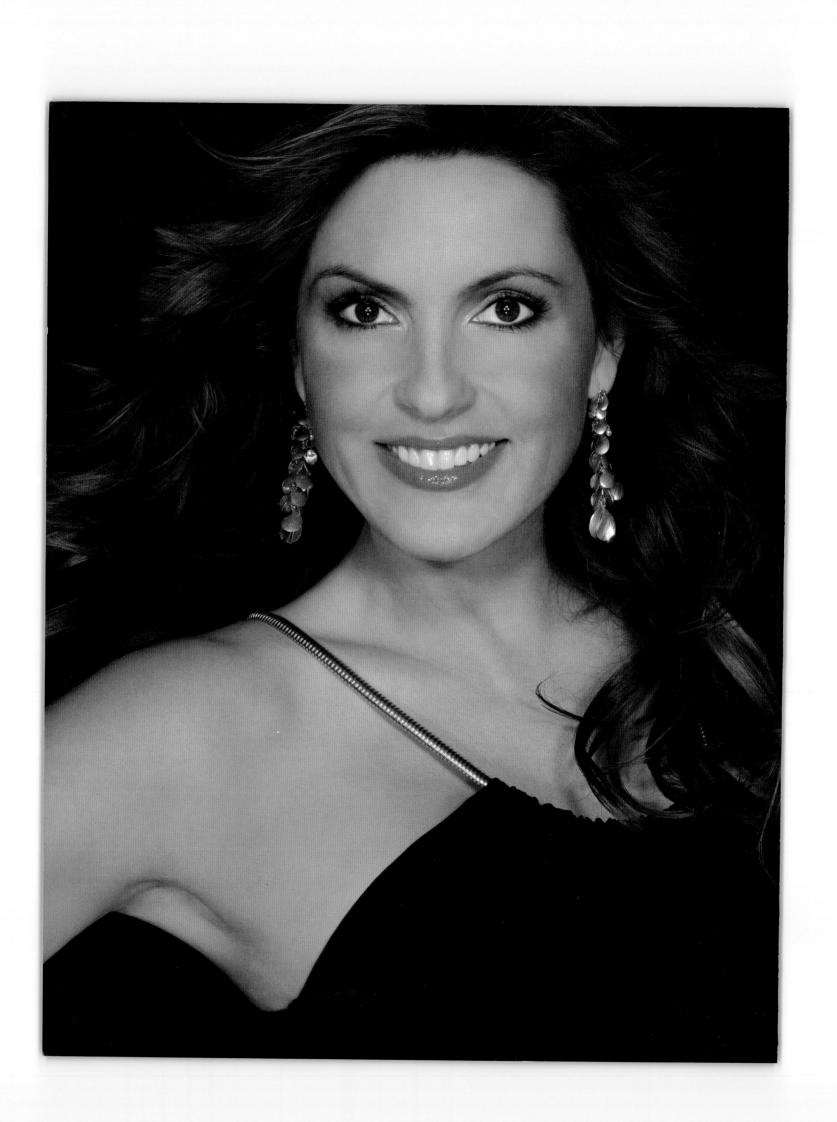

Mariska Hargitay ★

Scott on Mariska

Mariska is an award-winning actress. She's also the president and founder of the Joyful Heart Foundation, an organization dedicated to providing support and encouragement to survivors of sexual assault. Joyful Heart is an apt name since I think Mariska is a most joyful, generous woman. With her megawatt smile, she's exudes a sense of warmth and confidence that give her real presence. But perhaps the most appealing thing about Mariska and what many people don't know about her is that *she is really funny!* She's got a killer sense of humor, which reveals itself through her constant stream of humorous anecdotes and her impeccable comic timing. Whenever I work with Mariska, I always know it's going to be a day of fun and laughter. As talented as she is in *Law & Order: Special Victim's Unit*, I keep hoping she gets more chances to do comedy. She actually appeared in a sitcom, *Can't Hurry Love*, for a short time, but I think the world has yet to discover Mariska the comedian. Maybe I should say stunt comedian, because Mariska is also fearless to the point of insisting she do all her own stunts on *Law &*

Order (much to the chagrin of her producers). She could probably do one hell of a pratfall and have us all in stitches! There's simply nothing shy or girly-girl about this gifted, versatile actress. Her courage, strength, and uplifting spirit have allowed Mariska to touch many lives, both on camera as a tough but empathetic New York City detective and off camera as a compassionate leader who endeavors to heal wounded souls. It just doesn't get any more beautiful than that.

> Whenever I work with Mariska, I always know it's going to be a day of fun and LAUGHTER.

Mariska on Scott and Her "Secrets" for Staying Beautiful

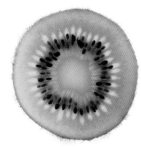

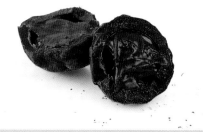

to replenish physically, just as much as we need to replenish spiritually and mentally. Plus, it'll be great for your skin.

● Eat well. This is an absolute must. I'm not saying you need to lunch at a five-star restaurant every day (especially in today's economy). It's about getting a balanced diet; you know the drill. For me, it's also about a little extra dark chocolate. They call it "the healthy chocolate." Seriously—a girl's gotta leave room for chocolate, right?! ● Listen to your body. Make sure you're finding the right balance of work, exercise, rest, and play. Your body will tell you what it needs; it's up to you to listen. But if it's saying, "Let's sit on the couch all day watching TV," tell it: "After we go the gym." ● Get in touch with your creative self. Start a journal, paint a picture, or grab your camera and take a walk. The best part is that you don't have to show it to anybody. Creative expression feeds your spirit, not some person looking over your shoulder, telling you to paint faster. ● Breathe. Take a moment, close your eyes, and just focus on your breath-

ing. In the midst of all the chaos, there's a calm, centered, healthy, joyful self in there that may just need a little air. ● Laugh. There's just nothing better for the soul. ● Finally, find your passion. Whether it's hang-gliding, antique books, karate, or volunteering your time... anything! I'm passionate about the Joyful Heart Foundation. It's an organization I started in 2004 to help survivors of sexual assault, domestic violence, and child abuse heal and reclaim their lives. Since then, more than 2,000 survivors have participated in our pioneering retreat and wellness programs. We reach thousands more with information on our website, and our participation in national educational and media awareness campaigns has planted the seeds of change in the lives of millions. But Joyful Heart isn't about affecting millions on a day-to-day basis. It's about touching the heart of the individual, one person at a time. I have seen the light go on again inside so many survivors. And it's those beautifully miraculous moments that keep me going in this work.

The work we do, the hearts we open, and the incredible people we encounter along the way—these are the roots of inspiration for me. So, find something for yourself that makes your heart joyful. That's how you make the most difference. And making a difference can lead to feeling good about who you are. It can give you confidence.

Confidence is beautiful. Compassion is beautiful. To have both with grace is beautiful. A person is beautiful when she has the courage to embrace her own potential and make choices for her life that are in sync with what's in her heart. And there's almost no bad hair day that a big smile and a little mascara can't fix! Although I do admit that there are those mornings when I wake up, look in the mirror, and think, "Man, I wish Scott Barnes were here to work his magic."

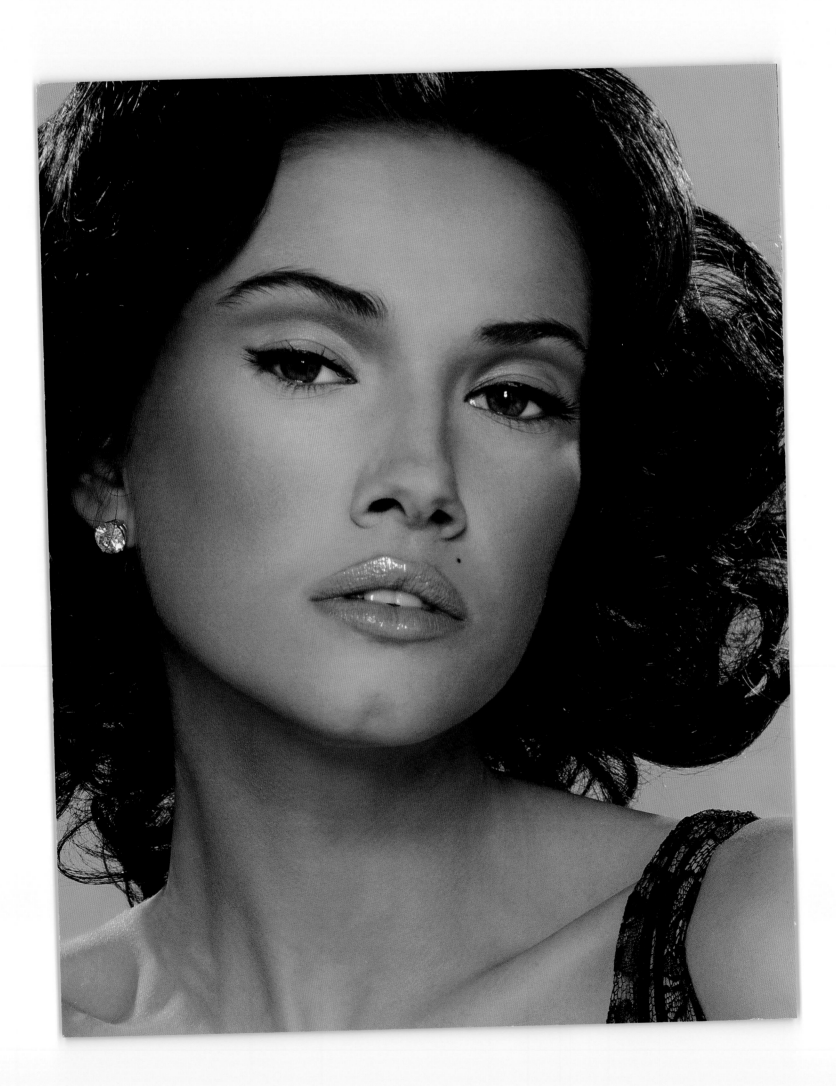

Nadiya:
Achieving That Sultry Look

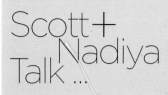

Nadiya is a long way from her roots. She's originally from Donick City, a small industrial town in the Ukraine that exports coal. She works full time as a print model and in TV commercials, but like the rest of the women in this book, Nadiya is more than just a pretty face. Having already seen much of the world, she has aspirations of moving into politics to help make a difference to those less fortunate in other parts of the world. She regularly volunteers her time at a local soup kitchen which she finds "inspiring" and that has given her a new appreciation for her own life.

When Nadiya walked into the studio, she immediately evoked the image of an Italian film siren—the kind of confident woman who exhibits passion and strength with a delicious femininity. I wanted to create a look for Nadiya that projected this same hot-blooded womanliness without overpowering her delicate features. By the time we were through, Nadiya smoldered with a look that could melt any man who crossed her path.

SCOTT: Do you normally wear makeup?
NADIYA: I normally use a little bit of makeup—usually some mascara, some black eyeliner, some lip gloss, a little bit of blush, and sometimes some under-eye concealer.

SCOTT: Do you think there's a difference between American women and Ukrainian women in their approach to beauty?
NADIYA: I think American women are more casual in their approach to beauty, but they display more taste than Russian women, who tend to overdo things.

SCOTT: Do you have a strict skin-care regimen?
NADIYA: Not really—except I use a French skin cream, Embryolisse, that I've been using for years. It's the best. I use it morning and night.

SCOTT: Do you have any beauty secrets?
NADIYA: Well, if I tell you it won't be a secret! I think the most important thing is to keep well hydrated and to exercise regularly.

(continued on page 77)

Creating Nadiya's Look

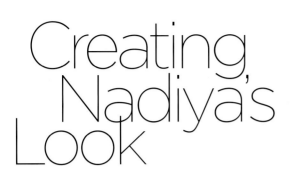

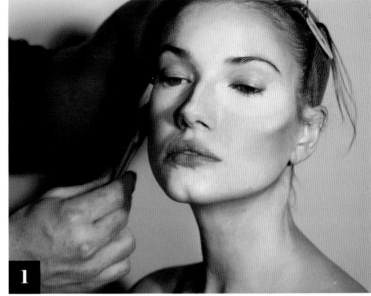

1

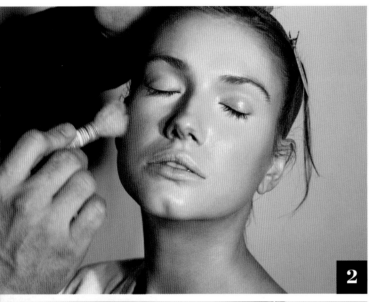

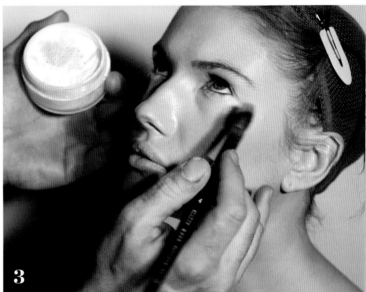

2

3

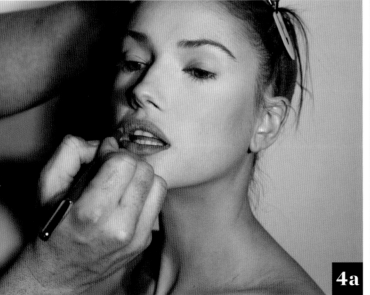

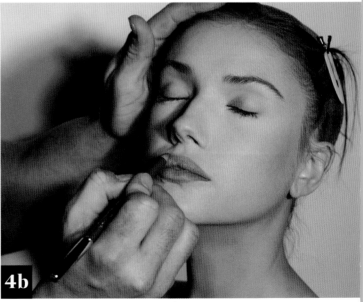

4a

4b

There's something feminine about the cleft in Nadiya's chin and her heart-shaped face. I wanted to give Nadiya a sultry look that would take her to the Isle of Capri. My decision to go in this direction actually had more to do with Nadiya's alluring demeanor than it did with her features.

1 Contouring, concealer, and foundation

Achieving a sultry look for Nadiya depends more on shading and highlighting to really sharpen and refine her delicate features. **(a)** Using light strokes with a goat hair brush, I applied contouring (dark) foundation: • Underneath the jaw line • Underneath the cheekbones • Down the sides of the nose • Underneath the tip of the nose • At the inner eye where the bridge of the nose meets the brow bone **(b)** Using a goat hair concealer brush, I applied highlighting (light) concealer using short brush strokes: • Under the eyes • Down the tip of the nose • In the middle of the forehead • At the center of the chin **(c)** Using a separate goat hair brush, I applied a thin layer of cream pale beige foundation all over her face, which I thoroughly blended with the contouring and highlighting for a smooth finish. *Remember: Effective application of contouring, highlighting, and foundation is about blending, blending, blending. Also, remember to apply some foundation underneath your chin and part way down your neck and blend thoroughly so there's no makeup line between your face and your neck, which is usually lighter than your face.*

2 Cheeks

Moving the blush brush in a circular motion, I blended a very pale flesh-tone peach cream blush on the apples of her cheeks. A darker blush would have looked too heavy with her dark hair.

3 Setting the look

With a very small concealer brush, I applied translucent powder in the following places to create an even, more porcelain-looking finish: • Under the eyes • On the side of the nostrils • On the top of the cheekbones

4 Lips

Nadiya had a nice full bottom lip and a slightly thinner top lip, so balancing out the lips and creating fuller lips overall required liner and lots of high gloss. **(a)** I followed Nadiya's lip line with a brown eyebrow pencil. For this particular look, I wanted a brown color that didn't have a lot of pink in it, but I also didn't want the harshness of a dark brown. **(b)** I finished her lips with pale pink gloss for a pouty, highly feminine look.

(continued from page 75)

SCOTT: And what do you do to stay in shape?
NADIYA: I like swimming. I like running. It's not that I go to the gym every day, but three or four times a week I try to get to the gym. Maybe I'm doing too much cardio, because I'm not very good at lifting weights. In the summer, I also ride my bike a lot. Now I want to try boxing. I've been into boxing since I was a young girl.

SCOTT: What is it about boxing that you like?
NADIYA: I think everybody thinks boxing is a very harsh sport, but what I like is that it's all about technique. It's a very smart game. It's a very interesting game that is about the way you have to move, from which corner you have to fight your partner. I like the strategy in it.

SCOTT: Is there anything you'd like to change about your look?
NADIYA: That's an interesting question. It really depends on the day. Some days I wake up and I like my face, but other days I wake up and I'm like, "Oh God..." There are many things I do and don't like about my face. It's strange about my face, because a lot of people say that my features are not

(continued on page 79)

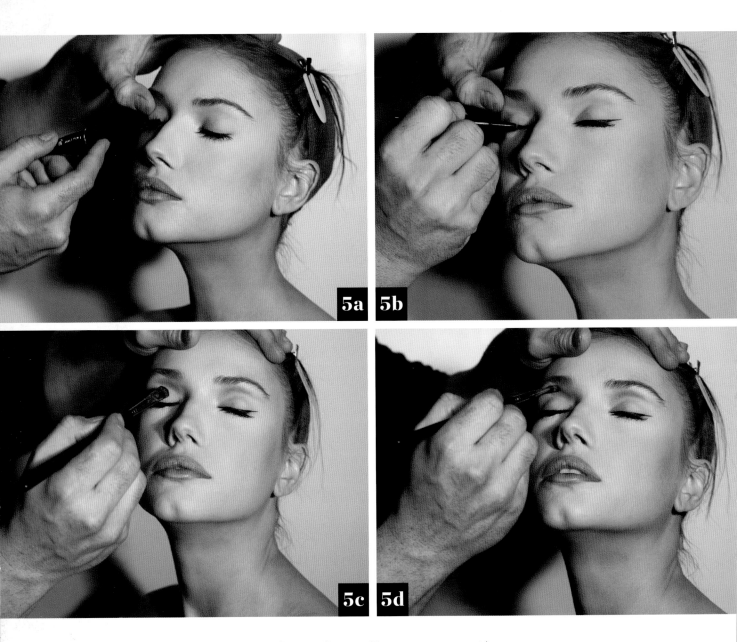

5a 5b
5c 5d

Tip When applying liquid eye liner, first remove the excess liquid on the palm of your hand (not on a tissue where it can pick up fibers). Then, wave the wand around a little so that it's not so wet; this gives you more control when applying the line, without applying excess color. If you mess up your liquid eyeliner...simply grab a Q-tip, lick it, and wipe away the liner. Saliva is the fastest (and cheapest) makeup corrector on the market!

I followed Nadiya's lip line with a BROWN EYEBROW PENCIL.

5 Eyes

This look was about creating a very "open eye," so I started with mascara. **(a)** I applied black mascara on the upper and lower lashes. **(b)** I curled Nadiya's lashes after applying the mascara since she told me her lashes were resistant to curling. So the mascara acted as a kind of gel to help hold the curl in place—a good trick for "styling" those hard-to-curl lashes. **(c)** I applied black liquid eyeliner to create a cat-eye effect. I drew a line across the top of her lid and extended the tail past the eye, making sure to keep it on an upward angle. The upward angle helps to lift the outside of the eye, creating a sexy cat-eye effect. I used a liquid eyeliner for Nadiya, instead of a pencil eyeliner, since liquid liners can provide a sharper, bolder effect as opposed to softer, smudgier pencils. **(d)** I applied a Smoky-Tan eye shadow above the normal crease in her eye to create more space on the lid. I used this color for a smokier, sexier effect on the eyes. Finally, I went back in with a beige eye shadow on the lid and on the brow bone so that it would give the effect of popping out these areas. Remember, light lifts.

Tip When lining your lips, feel free to use what you can find. You can certainly use a lip liner. Sometimes, you might find a color you like, but the pencil might be labeled as an "eyebrow pencil." You can still use it for lining your lips. In fact, eyebrow pencils have a bit more staying power because they have a denser consistency.

(continued from page 77)

quite perfect. And it's true—when you look at me, you see that one side of my face is a little bit different than the other side of my face. I think the right side is skinnier and the left side is puffier. But I don't want to change anything. I like the way I am. Obviously, I'm not perfect, but I'm doing my best to keep my body in shape and my skin looking good.

SCOTT: Are there other things you're passionate about?
NADIYA: I'm passionate about traveling and living life without worrying too much about whether the things you wish for come to you. Because life is too short, you have to try to be positive and not get too stressed. We have only one life, and we've got to try to do our best. If you really want something in life and you believe very strongly, maybe not today, not tomorrow, but it will happen to you.

SCOTT: Is there something you want strongly for yourself?
NADIYA: Yes, there are so many things. Sometimes I wish for very simple things: having a good family, a nice house with kids and dogs, and to be happy and healthy. But I'd like to go back to

(continued on page 81)

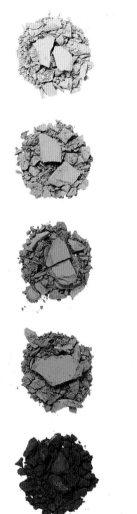

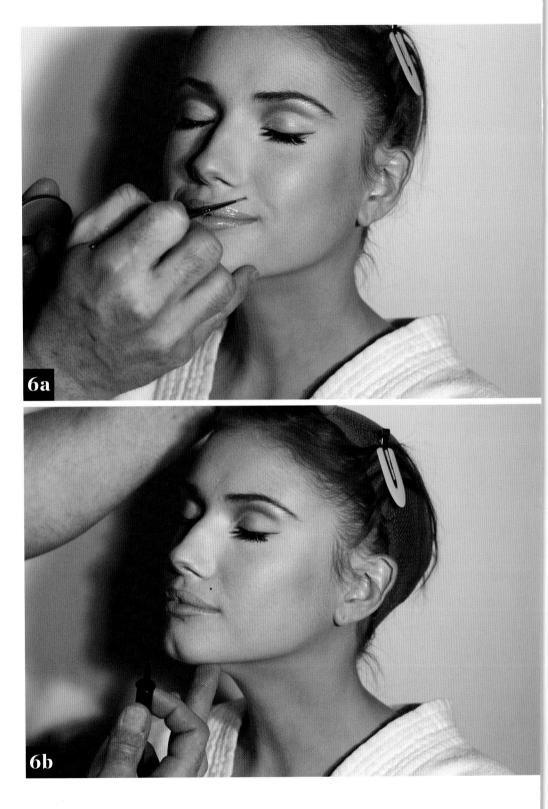

6a

6b

By the time we were through, Nadiya smoldered with a look that **could melt any man** who crossed her path.

(continued from page 79)

6 Completing the look

For the fun of it, I decided to give Nadiya a beauty mark just above her lips. **(a)** Just above her lips I applied a small dot using the black liquid eyeliner. **(b)** I then went back over the dot with the smoky tan eye shadow I used for her eyes to help set the liner and give the beauty mark a more natural look. I used a small pointed brush that is normally used for applying a eyeliner.

Tip When creating a beauty mark, never just put a black spot on your face because it will look like a black spot on your face. This is a two-step process. Go back over it after it dries with a brown eye shadow to cover it. This softens the harshness of the black and doesn't make it look like you have dirt on your face.

school to study political science. I would like to go into politics.

SCOTT: Why politics?
NADIYA: I recently started going to this soup kitchen, the Food Bank in Harlem. I was helping by cooking and serving food for homeless people. It is very hard work, and at the end of the day, you realize you have a good life with family and a good job these people just don't have. It's a very sad scene, even for the people who stand there ten hours a day trying to help these homeless people. These people who work at the Food Bank—the chef and the other people who help prepare and deliver the food—they work so hard. I found it very inspiring and decided that I also want to help people, but in a bigger way. I have traveled and seen much of the world. I see so many people in the world less fortunate than people in the U.S. when it comes to human rights. I would like to help make a difference somehow with all of that. I think we all have a responsibility to help each other.

REACTIONS...

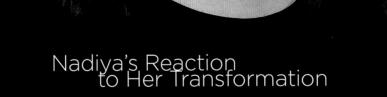

Nadiya's Reaction to Her Transformation

"I have never seen any other makeup artist do what Scott does, and I've worked with a lot of makeup artists. So, I was extremely surprised. For example, it's very impressive the way he starts working on your face. He does a mask first and then a face massage. I was most impressed with the way Scott does the skin. It's very interesting the way he applies the base; he has such a different technique. The French are always talking about how

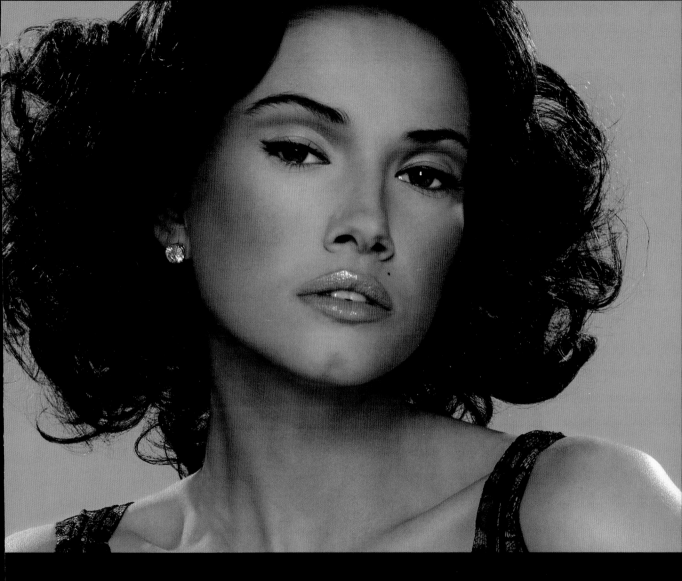

you should start with a good base: the skin. And Scott has a way
of covering up all the imperfections of the skin before starting
to apply the makeup. I now know how to make my skin look like
porcelain when I want this kind of look. Really, Scott showed me
just how far I could go with my makeup to create a different 'me.'
Much further than I ever realized."

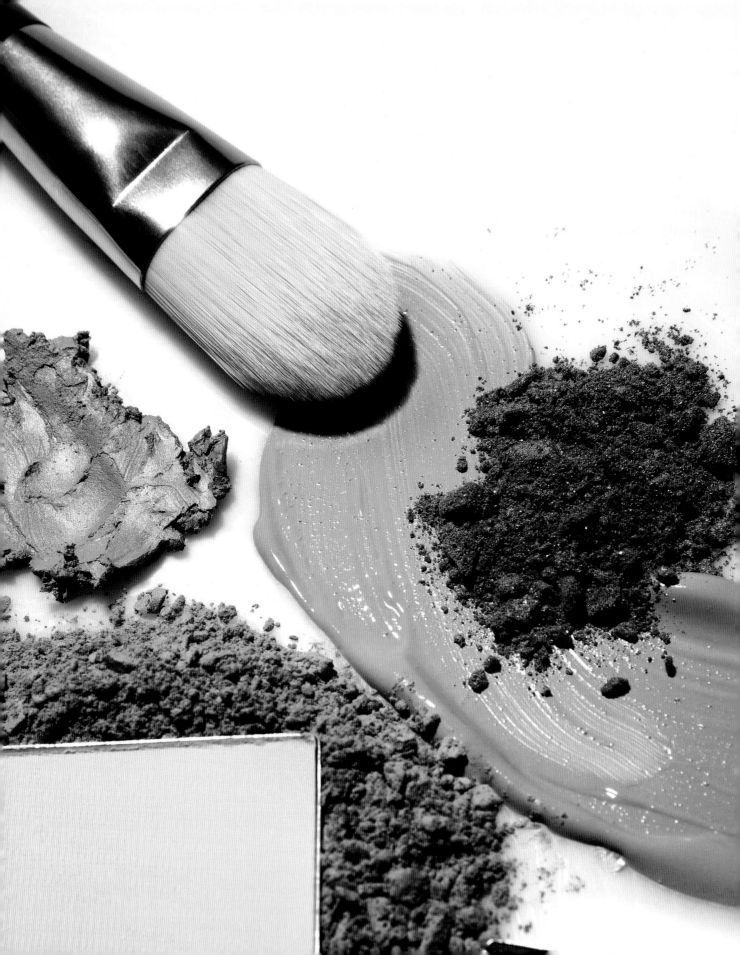

Breaking it Down

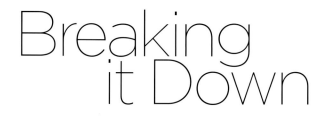

People approach makeup application with different degrees of experience. The trick is to not be afraid of it. It's only makeup; it washes off. Always feel free to make mistakes.

My aim with this chapter is to provide you with makeup application guidelines and tips based on many years of experience in the industry. It's impossible to cover everything in one chapter, so I'll address those things I feel make the biggest difference for achieving the best possible results.

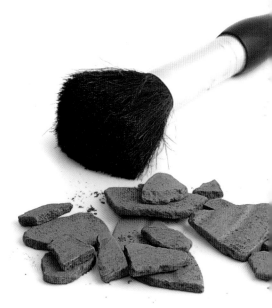

The finer the brush bristles, the smoother your makeup will go on.

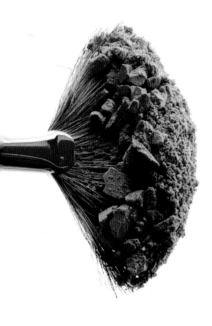

Brushes

Everyone has her preferred method of makeup application. Some people use sponges, some use fingers, and others use cotton balls and Q-tips. I use brushes. I believe brushes offer the ability to move the makeup around the face in a more fluid manner, as well as giving me more control in makeup application, which results in the smoothest blending possible.

I use brushes for every kind of makeup: cream, powder, and liquid. There is a misconception that brushes are best used for powder. But if you're using a brush with high quality bristles, it moves the makeup around just as well as any sponge will. It also effectively blends the makeup into the skin, instead of resting on top of the skin.

I could write a whole book on brushes, since there are so many different kinds. But who wants to read a book about makeup brushes? Instead of covering every kind of brush on the planet, here are some rules of thumb: ● Natural-hair makeup brushes (with bristles made from sable, squirrel, goat, or pony hair) are often much finer and softer and pick up makeup more easily than most synthetic (nylon or polyester) brushes, which are usually courser and stronger.
● Natural-hair brushes are best used for powders; synthetic brushes are best used for cream or water-based products. ● Brushes need some loving at least once a month. That means washing them thoroughly with soap and water. Baby shampoo works well. This can help extend the life of your brush for years. Also, when drying, be sure to lay your brushes flat so the water doesn't drip down into the ferrule and loosen the glue holding the bristles in place. Loose glue makes for shedding bristles. ● Brushes vary in price, from inexpensive ($8 to $15) to expensive, "professional-grade" ($20 to $50) brushes. Obviously, the more expensive the brush, the higher in quality the materials and craftsmanship will be when it comes to the bristles, the brush handle, and the way the bristles are wrapped for minimal bristle loss over time.

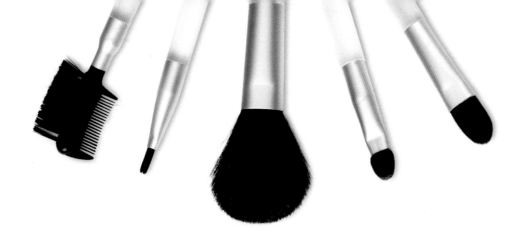

With that in mind, you may be asking, "Are expensive brushes really worth the additional money?"

You bet they are. If you want to achieve the highest-quality look, you've got to care about how you're applying your makeup. Blending and details matter. The finer the brush bristles, the smoother your makeup will go on. Streaky, cakey makeup is not pretty! Also, you'll save yourself time and money in the long run by not having to continually replace cheap brushes.

You can always build your set one brush at a time after you've got your basic brushes, which should consist of the following:
• Tapered contouring brush • Small concealer brush • Foundation brush • Blush brush • Large powder brush for applying translucent powder

Here are some additional brushes worth investing in: • Highlighter brush (looks like a fan) for applying shimmer highlight to cheekbones • Three eye shadow brushes: the largest for applying the base eye color, a smaller brush for applying color in the crease, and a thin chiseled brush for applying a line of shadow around the rim of the eye • Angled brow brush

I could go on and on about different brushes and their uses. I love brushes and so should you. A good brush can take you places, and it's worth spending a little time shopping for them and learning about all the different kinds available. I suggest hitting a makeup counter on a weekday afternoon when business is slow and asking one of those friendly makeup experts to demonstrate all the different brushes. Most of them are usually excited to offer advice and demonstrate various application techniques.

Good brushes, like good makeup, are worth the investment. Remember, you're worth it!

Some More Essentials

Creating your most beautiful self doesn't require a lot of makeup. It's more about good makeup application and having the right equipment. So, before you splurge on the latest eye colors or lipsticks, make sure you've got these essentials:

Airbrush and liquid foundation	No longer just for commercial artists and illustrators, this is a terrific application tool to have in your arsenal. You can apply a very thin layer of liquid foundation. They're worth the money (approx. $200) to achieve an even, feels-like-no-makeup coverage.
Blushes (2)	You should have one cream and one powder blush. Make sure at least one of them is a natural-looking color (soft rose or peach tones usually work best). The other color can be something bolder, more dramatic. You can always expand from there.
Brushes (5)	This is my tool of choice for makeup application, as discussed earlier.
Cigarette lighter	Have this on hand for warming your Maybelline eyeliner pencil (more on this later).
Contouring foundation	Contouring with makeup is cheaper than plastic surgery.
Eye drops	An eye solution such as Naphcon-A is great for removing redness from your eyes, as well as for masking red spots such as pimples.
Eye shadows (6 colors)	Brown, black, smoky gray, beige, mustardy yellow, and burgundy are great colors that work on everybody's skin and are best for achieving a more natural look. Like blush, you can always expand your color palette.
Eye pencils (2)	You should have one black and one brown eye pencil. I use Maybelline pencils. They're classic pencils that can be used in several different ways.
Eyebrow razor and a mini comb	The razor is invaluable for trimming eyebrows and removing facial hair. The mini comb can be any fine-toothed comb sized for use in small areas, such as an eyelash or mustache comb.
False-eyelash adhesive	Without this you would have to staple on your false eyelashes, and that gets messy! The brand I prefer is Duo.

Eyelash curler	Shu Uemura is the best eyelash curler on the planet. It costs a little more—about $18—but it's worth every penny. This curler is a bit wider and less curved, so it fits more eye shapes. It works particularly well on Asian eyes.
Facial moisturizer, light	It's always a good idea to moisturize before applying makeup. This helps to soften your skin and get rid of any dry patches.
False eyelashes (2 pair)	This is one of my favorite ways to add drama. They come as individual lashes or in strips. Have fun and experiment!
Foundation	For everyday, be sure to have foundation that matches your natural skin tone. A shade darker or lighter should be used for creating a particular look. Also, don't be afraid to mix two colors of foundation for a better match to your skin. (See "Applying Foundation" below for more on color selection.)
Highlighting concealer	This is one of the secret ingredients for creating the "glow"
Hydrating mask	This is good for moisturizing prior to makeup application.
Lip liner	A nude or flesh tone, something in line with your natural lip color, works best for just about everyone.
Luminizing mist	This helps you achieve that glow of young skin.
Mascara	Black is always better than brown; otherwise, what's the point?
Powder puffs	Powder puffs are great for pressing translucent powder into the skin and setting your foundation and blush.
Sheer lip gloss	Use gloss as a quick and easy way to freshen up your look. It's never out of style since moist, shiny lips are always sexy!
Shimmer highlight	For use on cheekbones, splurge on the good stuff. A little bit goes a long way, so it will last you awhile.
Translucent powder	This is good for all skin colors. Translucent literally means "through which light passes."
Tweezers	Tweezers are a necessity for plucking those evil little stragglers.

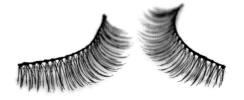

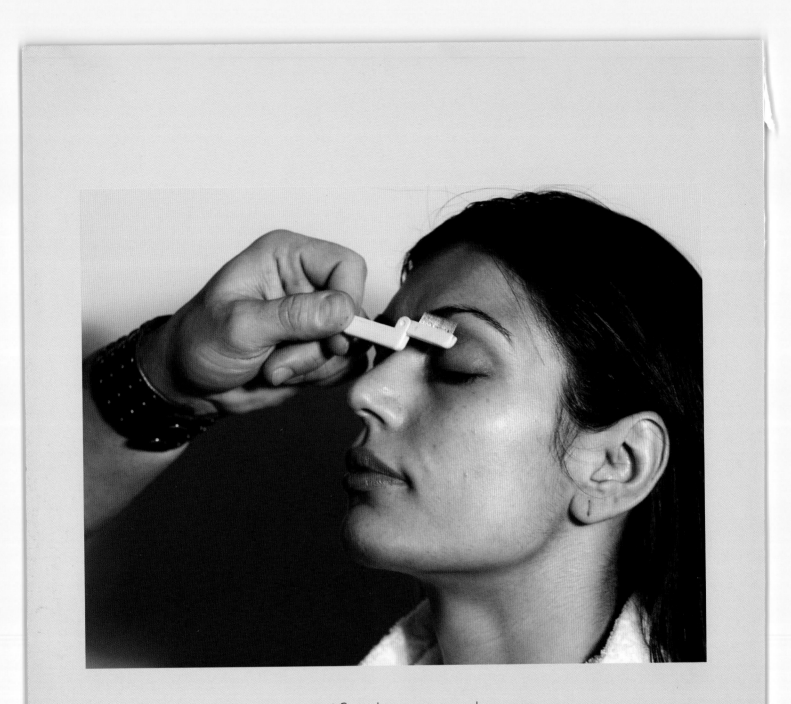

Lift the eyebrow
with the MINI COMB
and turn in the opposite
direction before trimming.

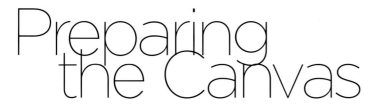

Preparing the Canvas

Before we get into some basics of makeup application, here are a few things you can do to prepare your face—the canvas—for the best possible results. You don't have to do these things on a daily basis, but the more attention you can give to prepping your face, the more remarkable the final picture will be.

Trimming and Shaping Your Eyebrows

Eyebrows are a prominent feature on the face—as prominent as the nose or lips—so be sure to give them some love.

For starters, make sure they're neat. I'm not an eyebrow fanatic. Some people get crazy about their eyebrows being perfect. I like it when they look more natural as opposed to perfectly manicured. Essentially, you want your eyebrows to lie flat on your face so they look smooth.

In addition to smoothing them down, you can also experiment with different shapes. But you want to be careful about how you do this. I recommend using a razor comb instead of tweezers for trimming and shaping. You can find razor combs everywhere, and they're cheap! To use a razor comb, follow these steps: **(1)** Put the mini comb in the hairs of the eyebrow **(2)** Turn the mini comb in the opposite direction to LIFT the brow hairs off the face. **(3)** Trim with razor. **(4)** Check the eyebrow by smoothing the hairs before trimming some more.

Remember to lift and trim the brow hairs little by little and check in between each trim to avoid cutting the brows too short.

Apply a tiny dab of gel or hair wax to help smooth down the brows after trimming.

The things I love about using a razor comb as opposed to plucking with tweezers are that you don't get ingrown hairs and if you decide you want to grow your brows back, you haven't taken out the follicle, which is what you do when you pluck. Once the follicle is removed, it takes much longer for the brow to grow back. Eyebrow styles change all the time, so give yourself the option of growing out your eyebrows and changing their shape. Remember the women from the 1950s? They plucked so much they couldn't grow their eyebrows back. I always say pluck as little as possible.

Many women end up with what I call "sperm brow" that clips up and then back around and looks like a little sperm whale. This has the effect of closing in your eye on the inside corner, because the brow nearest your nose is too heavy. Not a pretty look! The idea is to shape your eyebrows so that you lift and open up the eyes. You can experiment with many different shapes to find what kind of look you prefer, especially if you're trimming and not tweezing.

Shaping Eyebrows with Wax

You can mold your eyebrows with wax instead of plucking with tweezers or trimming with a razor comb. I use Geisha wax. Since your eyebrows naturally grow down from the top and up from the bottom of the brow, you can make them narrower by pulling them up with wax. It's good to do this when you're in the transitional phase of trying to grow out your brows for a new shape.

Tip If you have red hair and you want to match your eyebrow color with your hair color, don't apply red or brown color to your brow, which usually tends to look too dark. Instead, add yellow to the brow, because that's all red hair is: a lot of gold in brown hair. Using yellow achieves a golden red eyebrow, which will look more natural than a brown eyebrow.

Addressing Facial Hair

The other thing you want to consider is the amount of facial hair you have on your face apart from your eyebrows. Whether we like it or not, our society has come to value clean, smooth skin on women. Men can usually get away with just about any kind of facial hair. But that's probably because they have other things to worry about, like receding hairlines. So, take a good look at yourself and see whether you have a significant amount of hair on your upper lip or on the sides of your face. If you have a mustache or sideburns or excessive fuzz on any part of your face, you should remove it in whatever way you feel most comfortable. I recommend using a razor comb, because it's a quick, cheap, easy way to groom.

Many Mediterranean and Middle Eastern women (e.g., Italian, Greek, and Persian) tend to have more hair on the sides of their face and upper lip. Many of them use electrolysis to get rid of the fuzz. But if you don't have money for electrolysis, I recommend just using a razor, because the hair doesn't grow back any thicker. (The idea that hair grows back thicker after shaving is an old wives' tale.) Also, a razor doesn't pull and stretch the skin like waxing does.

The goal is to keep your face as hair-free as possible so you have a smooth, porcelain-like surface on which to apply your makeup.

Electrolysis can be very costly and very painful, but it's a permanent solution, as is laser hair removal. For laser removal to work, you have to have fair skin and dark hair; otherwise, the laser will burn you and you'll walk out with blisters since the laser doesn't register the hair as well and takes longer to zap the follicle.

If waxing is the route you choose to go, make sure you go to a good waxer, preferably someone who is recommended to you. Problems such as stretched skin, wax burn, or a skin rash can result if you use someone who isn't an expert waxer. So, don't be afraid to ask your friends for a referral. A bad waxer can do more damage, and it's just not worth the risk.

Removing Redness in the Skin

If you're dealing with a pimple or a breakout, apply a couple of eye drops to the irritated spot. This will reduce the redness a little, which makes the spot easier to cover with makeup. But it's not an acne killer. It simply constricts the blood vessels as it would in your eyes. Remember, this is a temporary fix. Be sure to speak to your dermatologist if you're experiencing red, blotchy skin or rosacea on a regular basis.

Also, yellow works wonders to combat redness. So, a foundation with a bit more of a peachy, yellowish tone works well for countering red skin.

Hydrating the Face

I often begin any makeover by applying a hydrating mask for ten minutes. It moisturizes the face, softens the eyes, and reduces any inflammation in the skin. If you don't have time for a mask, you can simply apply some light moisturizer and then wait a couple of minutes for the skin to absorb it before applying your makeup. Light moisturizing is an important step since it balances your skin for more even makeup application. Feel free to hydrate as often as once a week.

Relaxing the Face: The Lymphatic Drain

I learned this little trick in Shiatsu school. Your scalp and face are connected right at the ears and the jaw. If you press on the ears and the jaw, it hurts like hell, but it relaxes all the muscles in your face. When you sleep, you clench your jaw; when you drive you tense your facial muscles from the stress. You want to get rid of that tension by relaxing the muscles in your face with a lymphatic drain. The best part is, you can do this yourself.

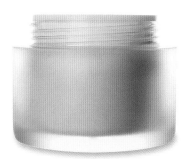

I do this with all my clients before red carpet events and photography sessions. It's especially effective after you've been flying. On a plane, the air is stale and you can't move around, so the blood doesn't circulate well throughout your body. A lymphatic drain helps drain the sinuses and gets your circulation going, which helps to oxygenate your skin. The results are amazing. A 40-year-old woman can have this process done and it will make her feel like she's thirty-five years old, just by pressing on both sides of her jaw! Now that's a trick worth learning, yes?

Taking a Moment

Once you're groomed, moisturized, and relaxed, you're well on your way to creating your most beautiful self.

But don't do anything just yet. Before applying any makeup, take a moment to appreciate the "you" without makeup. Notice your eye color, the shape of your lips, your nose, and each and every wrinkle. And as you study your face, fall in love with your features by reminding yourself that they are uniquely yours. Nobody else has the exact same arrangement of features, bone structure, or skin type as you have. Take a few deep breaths. Inhale the beauty of "self." Try to stay focused on the beauty of your individuality, not on your imperfections.

Also, take this time to get a cool, refreshing glass of water. As a general rule, most of us don't drink enough water, so try to get in the habit of using your makeup time as a time to hydrate your body and moisturize from within.

Once you've taken a couple of minutes to give yourself some love, you're ready to begin applying makeup.

Makeup Application

Step into the Light

Lighting is very important when putting on makeup. Be sure to apply your makeup in a well-lit area. That means making sure you have light on both sides of your face. Applying your makeup in front of a window for more natural light is a good idea, only if you aren't being hit by direct sunlight. The reason for this is that in direct sunlight, you tend to put on more makeup to compensate for the intensity of the light. Sunlight is wicked intense light—the most powerful light we have, in fact—and it simply can't be replicated with florescent lighting or 100-watt bulbs. So, you run the risk of looking like a crazy lady with too much makeup. Softer, natural light, similar to a slightly overcast day, is the ideal natural light by which to apply makeup. If possible, check your makeup in a couple of different mirrors with different lighting before walking out the door.

My favorite lighting for makeup application is a halogen bulb. I recommend picking up two cheap halogen lamps for your bathroom or vanity table. Just make sure the light doesn't come from below your chin, since that creates weird monster lighting and you'll end up looking like Boris Karloff. The light should be at the same height as your eye line for the best results.

Blend, Blend, Blend

I can't overemphasize the importance of blending. You'll see the word throughout this book, because it makes all the difference in good makeup application.

The point of blending is to make sure your makeup isn't sitting on top of your skin. You want the makeup to blend in with the natural fluids in your skin.

Want a smooth, flawless finish? Blend, blend, blend!

The best blending is achieved by moving your brush in a soft, circular motion, which helps to avoid lines on your face.

Creating a Smooth Canvas

APPLYING CONCEALER AND CONTOURING

You want to "build the face" by applying concealer and contouring. This is always the first step in the process before applying color makeup. But it's not about just flattening everything. It's about creating dimension, which is why you contour as well as conceal. Think of it as creating your canvas, which is all about defining your facial bones. Even if your bones are not prominent, you can use contouring and concealer to draw them out more by creating greater contrast in your face.

The rule of thumb for contouring and concealer is as follows: *Light adds to and dark takes away.*

Ultimately, you want to bring light to the center of your face. This kind of "glow" helps draw focus to the darker, more colorful features on your face—the eyes, brows, and mouth.

SELECTING YOUR CONTOURING AND HIGHLIGHTING COLORS

The general rule of thumb for selecting foundation for contouring and highlighting is as follows: go one to two shades darker than your normal skin tone for your contouring makeup and one to two shades lighter for highlighting makeup.

It's hard to get any more specific than this because it all depends on the amount of contouring and highlighting you want to do and how dramatic you want the effect to be. You'll see me vary the amount of highlighting and contouring on each woman, depending upon what I felt necessary for their particular look.

Also, I oftentimes use a light cream concealer as a way of creating the highlights when "building the face" in the beginning. Cream concealer has a slightly heavier consistency than that of powder or liquid foundation, which means it has the added advantage of providing more coverage. So, it depends on the amount of coverage you desire as to whether you decide to work with powder-, liquid-, or cream-based makeup for your contouring and highlighting.

APPLYING FOUNDATION

I prefer cream foundation over liquid foundation because cream-based makeup has more mobility—I can move it around more easily and with more control. Ultimately, you should use a foundation that you feel most comfortable with and that you feel works best with your skin. As a general rule, the consistency of cream foundations are good to use if you want more coverage; liquid and powder foundations tend to provide lighter coverage.

When applying your foundation, use a small amount and move your brush in a circular motion, blending all the while. If you're using a cream foundation, simply dip the brush directly into the makeup vial. If you're using a liquid or powder foundation, pour a small amount of foundation in the palm of your hand and dip the brush from there. *Remember, always wash your hands before applying makeup.*

Also, the neck and the face should know each other. So, be sure to take your foundation all the way down your neck. Why stop at the face when you can do your whole body! (Okay, maybe not your WHOLE body...but at least further down to make sure you include the neck.)

Again, the most important thing to remember about applying contouring, concealer, and foundation is that you don't want people to see it when you leave the house. Blend!

Selecting your foundation color

There are many different options when choosing your foundation color, so it can be a little overwhelming. But choosing the right color is easier than you think: simply match your foundation color to the color of skin on your collar bone or chest, not on your neck. Your neck is lighter skin than your everyday coloring because it is constantly protected from sunlight by your chin.

APPLYING BLUSH

Cream blush is always better if you have combination skin or you have dry patches on your face because the color in a cream blush will adhere more consistently across the apples of your cheeks, even if the skin texture isn't consistent. Powder blush, on the other hand, is better for more even-toned, normal skin. On oilier skin or combination skin, powder blush will adhere where the oily spots are and will collect around the dry areas of your face; as a result, you'll wind up with very uneven, blotchy cheeks that don't look smooth. And that's not sexy.

I often see women use blush for contouring underneath the cheeks, instead of using blush to add a touch of color to the cheeks. I say that if you want to contour and create cheekbones, use contour foundation! Otherwise, you look like you're from the 1980s when you put blush underneath the cheekbone.

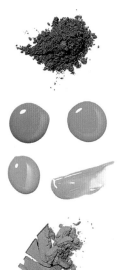

When you get flush, you're blushing from underneath. You want to mimic this natural blush when putting on your makeup. So, blend your blush onto the apples of your cheeks and up toward your temple a bit. This is particularly important for women over forty-five. If you apply your blush under your cheekbones, it's just going to draw your face down, and you'll come out looking too gaunt. The idea is to add youth, not age, to your face. And the easiest way to find the apples of your cheeks? Just smile!

ADDING SHIMMER HIGHLIGHTS

Whether or not you have prominent cheekbones, I still recommend highlighting them. The light will help draw the eye to this area and has the effect of "lifting" the face. In the transformations, you can see where I tend to consistently add highlights. Another good way think of it is to touch those "high" spots on your face where light first hits: the nose, the cheekbones, and the forehead.

ACHIEVING A BRONZY LOOK

Everyone feels better with a bit of color. If you are going after the sun-kissed look, start with a very light amount of bronzing powder on your brush and blend in a circular motion for the most natural-looking, warm glow. Build up your bronze slowly by layering. You can always add more, which is easier than trying to remove it. Look to Jessica Murphy's transformation into a bronze goddess for more tips on how to achieve the best fake tan!

Setting Your Makeup

Setting your makeup with translucent powder is an important step in the process that bears emphasis here. If you're going to go to all the work of applying foundation and blush, why would you want it to smear or look greasy? You can also put translucent powder on the eyelids and in the T-zone, before adding eye color, if you want to create "light" in those areas by mimicking the natural, lighter skin tone of those areas on the face.

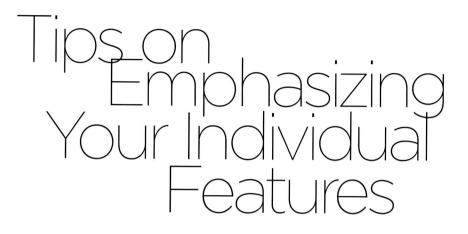

Tips on Emphasizing Your Individual Features

The point to remember with makeup application is that you don't want to try to emphasize all features at once. Instead, pick one feature you would like to highlight, and then go for it. If you're stuck in the same old way of doing things—if you normally emphasize your eyes, for instance—change it up a little and go for more dramatic lipstick and less eye makeup. You might be surprised how such a simple shift from one feature to another can dramatically change your look.

Lips

Women sometimes think they can get away wearing nothing on their lips, particularly during the day when going for a more natural look. But it's still important to wear something on your lips, even if it's only a clear gloss or lip balm, to help keep the lips moisturized and protected. Otherwise, you'll find yourself licking your lips a lot, which actually results in dry, cracked lips. Not sexy! Lipstick also helps a woman look more "put together," and even "kissable." And what woman doesn't want that?

LINING THE LIPS

Lining your lips is a useful trick for balancing out the lips (e.g. if your upper lip is thinner than the bottom lip) or if you want to make the lips appear fuller than they really are.

When lining the lips, the idea is not to create a hard line, but rather to provide some definition for the mouth. So, it's better to go with a light touch when lining to provide a more natural look.

Always be sure to line directly on the lip border or just inside it, but never outside the lips; otherwise, you will look like that crazy lady at the mall. And make sure after applying that you softly blend the liner, so you avoid ring-around-the-mouth.

It's important to use a nude or flesh tone lip liner when going for a more natural look. For other colors, it's best to either match your lip liner to your lipstick color or go only one shade darker than your lipstick color, as a general rule of thumb.

Creating Fuller Lips

To create fuller lips, draw straight across the peak on your upper lip, without emphasizing the dip in the center. This creates the illusion that your lips are fuller with that come-to-me pouty look. That's very sexy, no? Be sure when drawing the line across, you don't go higher than the two peaks with the line; otherwise, it will look as if you lined above your natural lip line.

REMOVING DRY SKIN FROM DRY LIPS

Everyone gets dry lips now and again. Luckily, it's easy to remove dry skin from your lips without causing irritation. Apply some lip balm to a mini makeup brush and gently scrub the brush back and forth on your lips to slough off the dead skin. In addition to getting rid of dry skin, you're also providing circulation to the lips, so the lips will appear plumper and with added color.

If you brush a little bit around the outside of the lips—gently—you can also get rid of any little blackheads that you might have from lip balm, lipstick, and so on.

You can use a toothbrush for this, but I recommend you buy a mini makeup brush with boar's hair bristles instead. These types of bristles have a little better give to them, so you're not destroying your lips.

Eyes

It's well known that "the eyes are the windows to the soul." We communicate so much of who we are and how we feel through our eyes. The eyes are the first feature we go to when greeting someone or when we want to know how the other person feels. Eyes are uniquely our own—no two pair are alike—and as you can see in these transformations, I believe eyes deserve special emphasis.

As you go through the book, you'll notice that I use certain colors to help bring out a particular model's distinct eye color. My recommendation is to play around with different color combinations to see which ones compliment your eyes best, using these transformations as a guideline. The trick is to draw out your own eye color as opposed to overshadowing your eyes (quite literally) with too much colored makeup. That usually means picking eye shadow colors that contrast

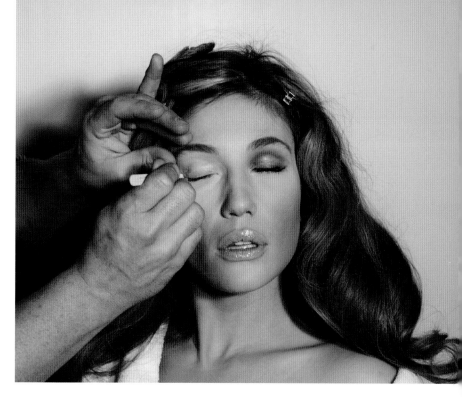

with your eye color, instead of trying to match the color of your eyes. (Of course, there are exceptions to this general rule too, depending on what look you're trying to achieve.)

These are some additional techniques you might find helpful when addressing certain types of challenges with your eyes:

EYES THAT ARE HOODED

Look in the mirror and stare straight ahead. If you see no eyelid on your eyes, you have hooded eyes. When applying eye shadow in this case, the last thing you want to do is put a light color on top of this kind of lid because that will make your eyes look puffier and more hooded. So, it's better to go with very minimal eye color and accentuate the eyes with mascara or fake eyelashes. Lauren Bedford's transformation is a good demonstration of this approach.

EYES THAT ARE TOO FAR APART

If you feel your eyes are too far apart, you can make them appear closer together by drawing the emphasis toward your inner eye. To do this, apply the heaviest portion of mascara or false lashes on the inside corner of your eyes to give the illusion that the eyes are closer together.

CLOSE-SET EYES

If you feel that your eyes are too close together, you can make them appear farther apart by drawing the emphasis toward your outer eye. To do that, apply the heaviest portion of mascara or false lashes on the outside corner to draw the eyes outward.

SMALL OR DEEP-SET EYES

If you have small eyes, put some white cream eye shadow on the inner corner of your eyelids to help open up your eyes. This technique is especially beneficial if you've got deep-set eyes. Oona Hart's transformation is a good example of how to make small eyes appear larger.

Effective Eye Lining with a Pencil

You can flatten out your eyeliner pencil and create an edge to it that allows you to go right up against the lid. I usually drop the pencil straight on the table. It's easier than using an eyeliner with a point, since it allows for a better angle on the pencil.

USING LIQUID EYELINER

Eyeliner has been used for decades to create a dramatic, glamorous effect. Proper application of liquid eyeliner is about removing excess liquid from the wand before applying.

Take the tip of the eyeliner and remove some of the liquid by drawing a couple of lines on the back of your hand. Then wave the eyeliner in the air to help it dry slightly before drawing on your eyelid.

Keep in mind that heavy eyeliner has the effect of closing up the eye. So, I don't necessarily recommend it if you're using false eyelashes. The whole point of the lashes is to create open, fluttery, flirty eyes. So, think twice before lining the eye as well.

If you do decide to use eyeliner with false eyelashes, be sure to draw all the way to the inner corner of the top eyelid with the liner so that the line doesn't stop short where the eyelashes stop.

Tip Sometimes leaving the eyes alone works best. In other words, let the color of your concealer come through on the eyelid instead of putting on eye shadow. You can always add some false eyelashes to accentuate your eyes, instead of covering your eyes in a lot of heavy color. Sometimes less is more.

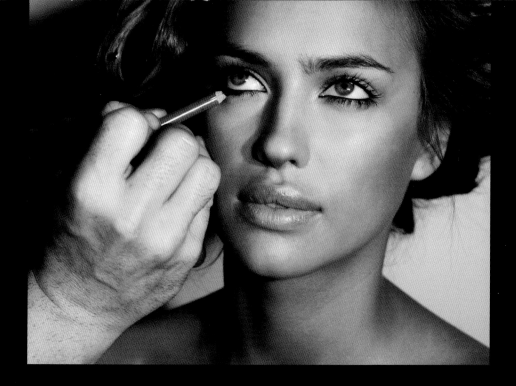

Working with a Maybelline Eye Pencil

A Maybelline eye pencil is my black pencil of choice. It is the blackest pencil I know. It's the least expensive pencil on the market and it can work both as an eyeliner and as an eyebrow pencil. But before you use it for lining your eyes, you first want to soften it; otherwise, it pulls on the skin due to its harder consistency and creates wrinkles, and who needs those? All you need is a cigarette lighter. Simply wave the tip of the pencil through the flame a couple of times to soften it.

Remember to blow on it and test it on your hand before putting it on your eye!

The consistency should be firm, to the point that it glides. It should not be wet, and you shouldn't be able to bend the tip. (If it goes on too soft, it will clump up in your eye and irritate it.) Once it cools down almost to the point of getting hard again, you can use it like a crayon, and the effect will be like a soft charcoal pencil.

APPLYING MASCARA

For really lush lashes, I recommend coloring both the underneath and the top of the lashes. To avoid clumpy lashes, lay the mascara brush at the base of the lashes, jiggle the brush from side to side, and then whisk it up through the rest of the lashes. This loads the mascara at the base of the lashes. It doesn't leave you with clumpy ends but still looks really thick and luscious.

As far as color goes, I use black mascara—always. What's the point of using anything but black? That's like saying, "Hi, I'm going to pretend like I'm putting mascara on, but I'm really not!" If you want people to see your eyes, black is the only way to go.

USING FALSE EYELASHES

I love false eyelashes. They're a great way to make your eyes look bigger and add drama. Just make sure you don't wait until an hour before your big event to learn how to apply them. It takes a little practice and patience to learn how to apply them so that they look natural.

When you use false eyelashes correctly, they never look "costumey." You can go heavy on the lash with a gown or a beautiful dress or a trench coat. If you use a heavier lash, just be sure not to overdo it by also applying a lot of eye shadow. Less is more in this case because you're picking one feature and you're taking it all the

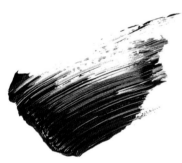

way there, which makes a bolder statement. It's better than adding a color on every part of the face. I get really tired of color, which is odd for a makeup artist to say.

Proper application

Make sure your lashes are clean before applying faux lashes, which adhere to both your eyelid and your natural eyelashes. It's a good idea to put the eyelashes up to your eye to see how long they are before adding adhesive. Sometimes you may need to trim the false eyelashes, if they look unnaturally long-unless, of course, you prefer to look like a drag queen.

Apply the adhesive to the strip of eyelashes (not to your eyelid) and set the lashes along your natural lash line. You have a few seconds to adjust the lashes as the glue begins to dry.

There are two types of eyelash adhesive: temporary and semi-permanent. Temporary lasts until you apply water to the adhesive. Semi-permanent can last up to five days.

Sometimes you might decide that demi lashes (half lashes) are all you need for opening up the eye, instead of a whole strip. You can cut the eyelash in half and apply either one or both halves to the outside or inside corner of your eye, depending on the look you want to create.

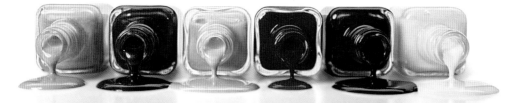

Proper removal

Use an oil-based remover to remove false eyelashes. Never pull the eyelashes off without using a remover; otherwise, you risk pulling and stretching your delicate eyelid skin. Treat your eyes with care!

Applying individual lashes

Individual lashes give you much more control over the look and feel of the lash. I often use individual lashes when I want to give a more open, airy feeling to the eye. Placement of individual lashes is key. Applying the lashes to the outside corner keeps the eye more open. Applying the lashes to the inside corner creates a more doe-eyed effect. Or you can apply them in different directions for a star-burst effect. Adhering individual lashes can be a little tricky at first, but they provide many more options once you get the hang of them.

Hands and Nails

Hands are a very feminine feature on a woman. Or at least they can be if they are well manicured. There's nothing tackier than a beautiful woman with dry hands and unkempt nails. Beautiful hands can actually turn a person on, so don't forget this important step when beautifying.

I always like it when the nails look clean and look like an extension of your hand. It's sexy. I don't like seeing really bright colors on long nails. I think too much red and pink on white skin pulls out the red in the skin. This emphasizes the redness on the knuckles and in the cuticles because red fingernails make whatever's red in your skin look even redder. If your nails are dressed with a more natural color, it makes for a better blend from hand to nail, and it elongates the fingers (So, this is a good point to remember if you've got short, stubby fingers!). A light beige polish looks great. A French manicure is always good.

There are some exceptions to the rule of natural color on long nails, though: ● **Women of color:** Women with really dark skin tones can pull off brighter colors without a problem. ● **Shorter nails:** If you want to sport shorter nails, some of the darker colors—burgundy, chocolate, black, navy—can be fun. So knock yourself out.

When in doubt, go without a color. But still moisturize your hands and make sure the nails are smooth and trimmed. Not only do beautiful hands look more feminine, they make you feel more feminine!

Of course, the same goes for feet. Don't subject everybody to rough heels and fungus toes. Get in the habit of treating your feet to a pedicure—either in home or at a salon—at least once a month to help address these issues. In the case of polish on toenails, go for color. Hot pink or red toenails are oh, so sexy!

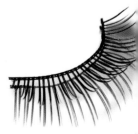

Trans*f*ormations

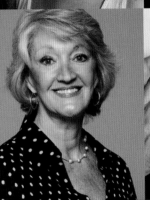
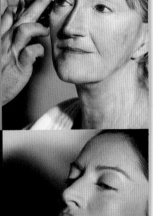
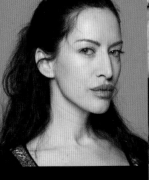
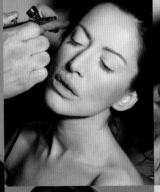
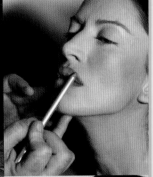
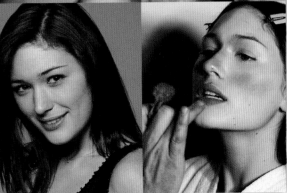

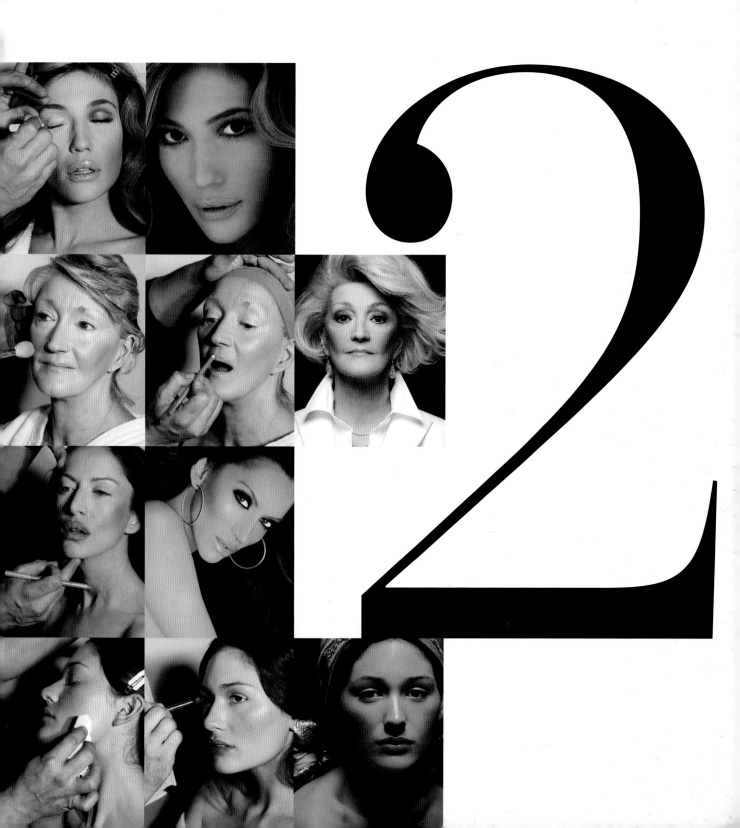

2

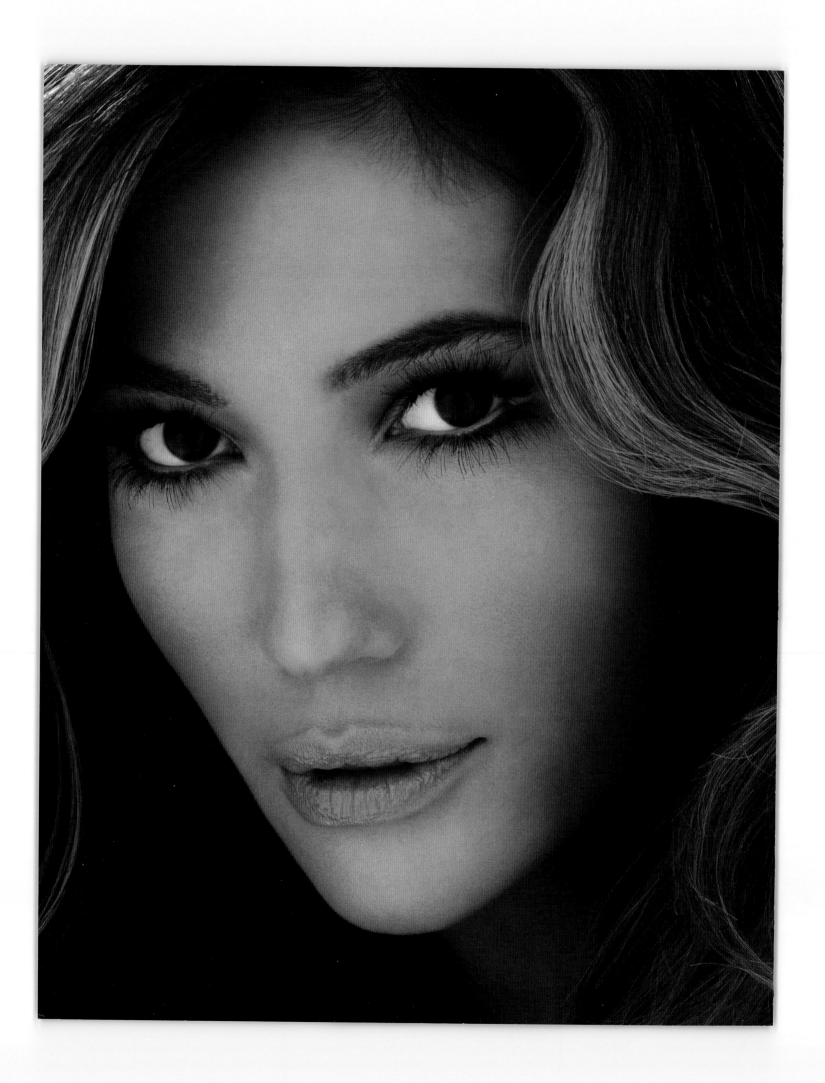

Oona:
Bringing Sensuality to the Forefront by Playing Up the Eyes

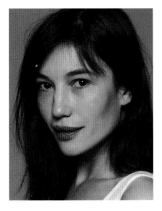

Oona is one smart cookie who isn't easily impressed. She lets her guard down slowly—not because she's apprehensive but because she doesn't need anybody telling her how to do things. She stays attuned to current events, and she has her opinions. Although Oona models, her world is not about her appearance. It's about her family—she's married with a two-year-old son—and her two passions: photography and painting.

Oona has warm, intelligent eyes that seemed to flirt with me when she spoke. Unfortunately, they were dwarfed by her more prominent cheekbones and mouth. I knew that once we shifted the focus to her enticing eyes, Oona's sensuality would come hurtling to the forefront. In the end, not only did Oona lose her cool demeanor, she became undeniably hot.

SCOTT: What is your typical morning beauty regimen?
OONA: I don't have a routine. I'm not really rigid about that sort of thing. Sometimes when I get up in the morning, I do nothing. If I'm going to work, I will wash my face and put moisturizer on. I wash my face before bed. Sometimes I use something cute and fancy and sometimes it's just a bar of soap in the shower. I use a heavy moisturizer at night usually, but not always.

SCOTT: Today you didn't come with much makeup on. Is that because you don't prefer to wear makeup?
OONA: I love makeup. I'm not somebody that wears it all the time—I don't feel naked without it—but I enjoy wearing it, like when I'm doing something festive. I think when I was younger I experimented more with makeup, but now I don't have the time as much as I used to because my son will come over and grab some eye shadow and run into the other room.

(continued on page 111)

Creating Oona's Look

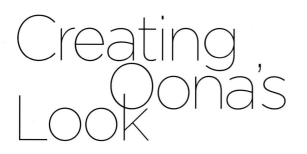

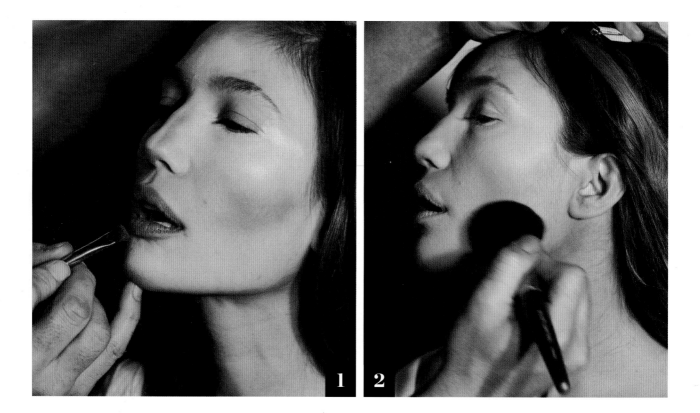

1

2

Tip When bronzing, make sure you leave the center of the face alone so that you don't darken it. Think of it as creating a diamond shape of light at the center of your face.

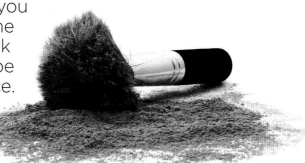

Oona exuded a sex appeal even when she was trying to downplay her beauty by wearing no makeup, beat-up jeans, boots, and a tank top. She has a combination of vulnerability, toughness, and sensuality, all the necessary ingredients for an explosion. Bombshell!

....

1 Contouring, highlighting, and foundation

Oona clearly has a prominent bone structure, so the contouring for her was minimal, more like adding a blush than creating a hollow. **(a)** Using a goat hair brush, I applied minimal contouring (dark) foundation: • Underneath the jaw line (slight contour) • Underneath the cheekbones • On the sides of the nose • At the temples • Under the tip of the nose (gives the illusion of shortening the nose) **(b)** Using a concealer brush, I applied highlighting (light) concealer: • On top of the cheekbones • Underneath the eyebrows • Under the eyes • On the bridge of the nose • At the center of the chin **(c)** Using a separate goat hair brush, I applied a thin layer of a very neutral beige foundation on top of the contouring and highlighting. *Remember: Blend thoroughly, moving the brush in a circular motion to marry all the colors together for a seamless transition.*

2 Setting the look

I finished off with a nice dusting of translucent powder for setting the makeup and providing a seamless finish. Using a small powder brush, I applied translucent powder: • On top of the cheekbones • Underneath the eyebrows • On the bridge of the nose • At the center of the chin

3 Bronzing

Using a large powder brush, I applied a pale bronzing powder, moving upward from the neck and jaw line to her cheeks and working the brush in a circular motion. This creates a very soft effect in the cheek area.

(continued from page 109)

SCOTT: Do you have any features you like or dislike?
OONA: I don't know if I have a specific feature, at least not one that you use makeup on! Sometimes I wake up and feel really good about the way I look, and other days I feel a little busted. But I think that's the same for everybody. No matter how glamorous I might look to somebody else, I have those days when I wake up and I feel great and those days I don't. But I don't really think about how I look every day, and if I did, I might be less satisfied. Maybe that's the trick: You just can't think about it too much, just an appropriate amount to have some self-respect. But not so much that you become too critical because anybody can overdo the self-criticism, which just doesn't do anybody any good.

SCOTT: How does a person avoid being overly critical of herself?
OONA: I think you have to like your life, and then a lot of things become beautiful.

SCOTT: What do you like to do for fun?
OONA: I have a kid, so I play with him. And I have a man, so I play with him too. My kid is two.

(continued on page 113)

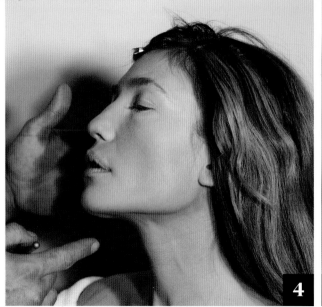

4

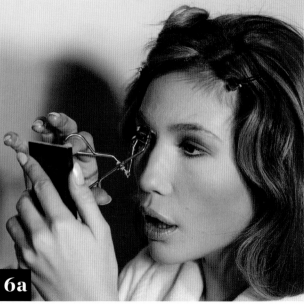

6a

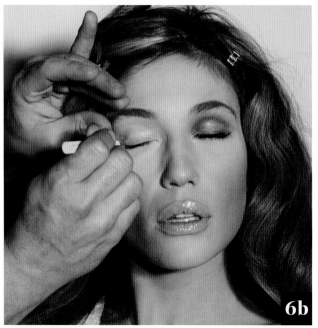

6b

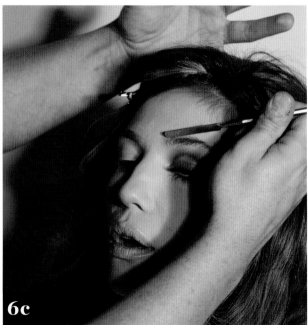

6c

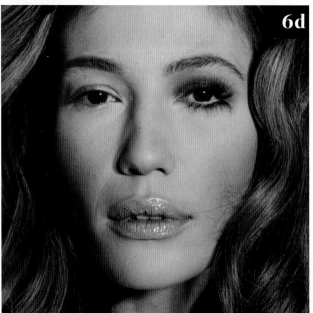

6d

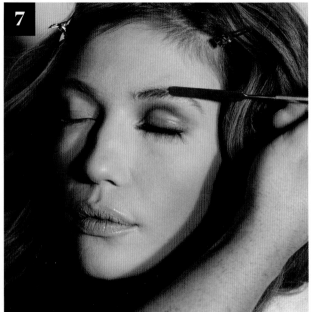

7

4 Cheeks

This look requires only a bronzing powder as a blush. So, I applied no blush whatsoever on Oona's cheeks.

5 Lips

I used a transparent shimmer gloss to accentuate Oona's mouth. Oona has very full lips, so no lip lining was necessary.

6 Eyes

To demonstrate the subtlety of the eye shadow, I finished one eye to show the effect it has on opening the eye. This is how it broke down: **(a)** I had Oona curl her own lashes. **(b)** I used just a splash of the bronzer for minimal covering on the whole lid. You want a light touch here to avoid putting on too much color and giving a heavy, over-tanned look. **(c)** I applied a basic chocolate-brown shadow from the lash line of the upper lid to just about above the crease. **(d)** I surrounded the rest of the eye with this same chocolate-brown shadow to create a lot of depth with a neutral tone. **(e)** I topped off the eye with individual false eyelashes on the upper and lower eyelids. I used individual lashes because I wanted the lashes to feel very fluffy, which you can't always achieve with a strip of false eyelashes. **(f)** The last thing I did was apply white eyeliner on the inside of her lower eyelid to help open up the eye. This gives the effect of creating a larger eyeball.

7 Eyebrows

I liked the shape of Oona's eyebrows, but they were just a bit furry for the furry lashes. So for minimal shaping, I opted to use stiff hair wax and a bit of hairspray. Here's what I did: **(a)** I applied the eyebrow wax on the brow with my fingers, sweeping upward.

(b) With a credit card, I pushed the eyebrow down and pinched the hairs together, creating a thinner brow without plucking.

Voilà! Thinner eyebrows!

Tip You can warm up your eyelash curler by rubbing the part you apply to the lashes back and forth between your fingers so that it works more like a curling iron.

(continued from page 111)

He tests his boundaries, but he's far from terrible. He's really amazing. Otherwise, I spend my time either painting or doing photography.

SCOTT: Where did the photography interests come from?
OONA: My dad's a photographer, and I grew up assisting him in the studio. I've been doing photography as long as I can remember. I photograph in the old-fashioned way because I learned those techniques from my dad. So, I prefer shooting with film and large-format cameras.

SCOTT: Are you strict with yourself when it comes to food and drink?
OONA: I don't eat meat. That's probably my only thing that's an absolute. I'm not a vegetarian. I eat fish, but I don't eat meat. And I eat fish because if I don't eat any meat, I can't really go anywhere exotic. By allowing myself to eat fish, I can usually get by.

SCOTT: What do you think it takes to be beautiful?
OONA: I think it's important to be happy. I think if you're happy, you can be happy with yourself, you can find other things encouraging and beautiful and positive, and you can be beautiful yourself.

REACTIONS...

Oona's Reaction to Her Transformation

"It was a huge transformation. I looked fantastic. No one had ever made me up exactly as Scott did. Every time you're made up, it's different, but I've never seen myself quite the same way before. My eyes were definitely more prominent. And I learned some great techniques. I've incorporated his eyebrow trick into my regular routine."

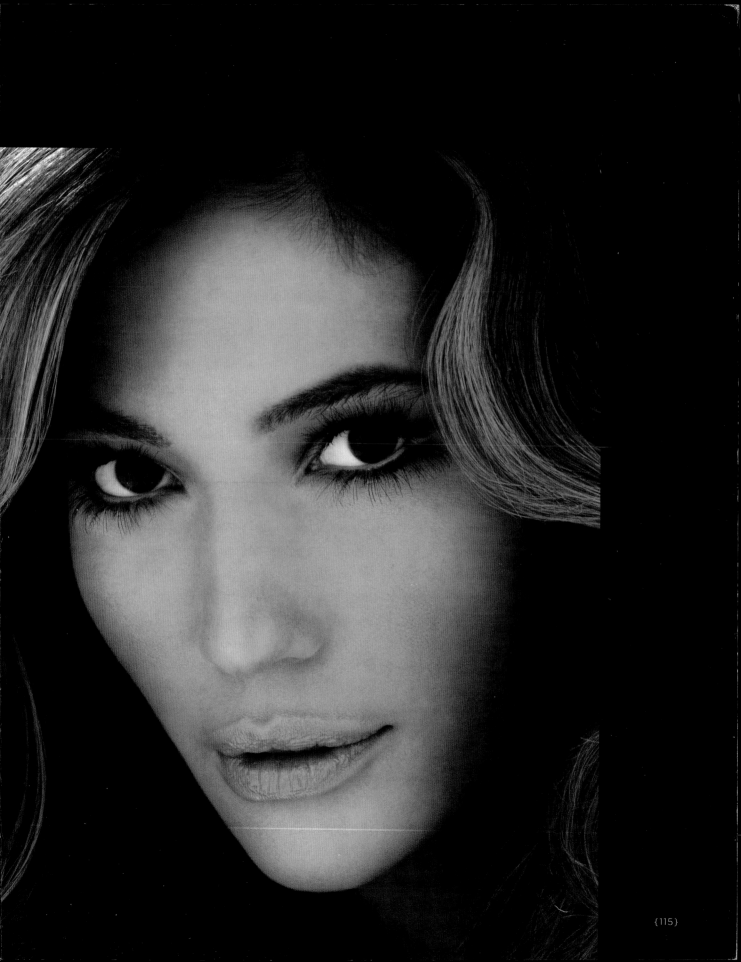

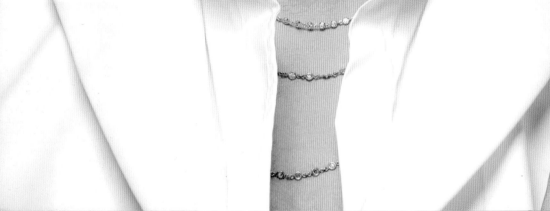

Elizabeth:
Using Airbrush Foundation for Added Radiance and Distinction

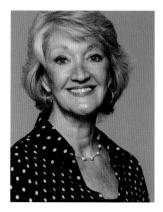

Elizabeth stopped teaching years ago, yet she's anything but retired. She continues to work as a substitute teacher, volunteers as a horseback riding instructor on weekends, stays actively involved in the lives of her three daughters, and spends as much time as possible with her five-year-old grandson. Oh, she also "does some movie and commercial work on the side." Elizabeth is a pro-age woman who believes in taking good care of herself and keeping up her appearance. Elizabeth has a naturally handsome countenance, and I was excited about enhancing her strong Irish features, particularly her sparkling emerald-green eyes. In the end, a more distinguished Elizabeth emerged with a new look that spans from city chic to equestrian elegance.

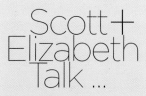

Scott + Elizabeth Talk ...

SCOTT: What's important to you in life?

ELIZABETH: My family— I have three daughters and a grandson, and I try to spend as much time with him as possible. We went ice skating recently—he loved that. And of course, we have fun in the park. We do whatever sounds like fun together.

SCOTT: Would you mind telling me your age?

ELIZABETH: I'd rather respond with the old cliché, "Age is just a number." It's how you feel, how you act, and how you think about things; that's what's important. I don't feel old, so why should I be saddled with a specific number so that people who don't know me will automatically dismiss me as being old and with outdated ideas? I know people who are old at forty, and I know others who are young at eighty. It's all in the mindset.

SCOTT: As a beautiful woman, how do you feel about getting older?

ELIZABETH: Let's face it: Aging is inevitable.

(continued on page 119)

Creating Elizabeth's Look

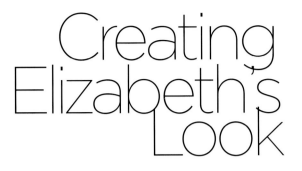

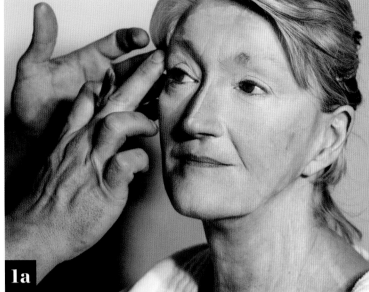

1a

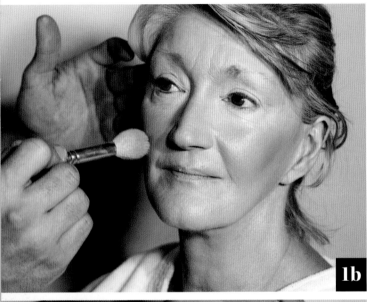

1b

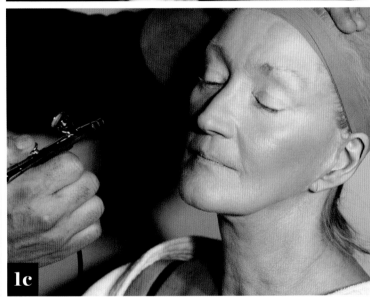

1c

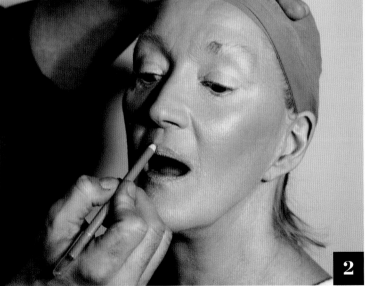

2

Tip When using an airbrush to apply foundation, it's very important to cover your hair, particularly if you're fair-haired. A bandana, a stocking cap, or even a hair band works—just something to pull the hair off your face and protect your hair from being covered in a mist of makeup!

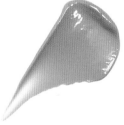

Elizabeth is a beautiful woman with a strong chin, nose, and eyes. She also has ruddy skin, which is not surprising since skin tone usually changes as we age. By emphasizing her strong points, I felt we could modernize Elizabeth's look to give her a more distinguished appearance.

1 Contouring, highlighting, and foundation

This was a very simple process with Elizabeth. I opted to use an airbrush to apply Elizabeth's foundation. Airbrushing has the effect of looking and feeling like there is virtually no makeup on the face. Heavier foundations on mature skin can sometimes make a person appear older, since the makeup often settles in the creases of the skin. I wanted to provide just enough foundation on Elizabeth to eliminate the redness in her skin but still even out her skin tone.

I had to put a stocking cap on Elizabeth's head, much to her chagrin. This ultimately prevented her extremely light hair from turning brown as a result of the makeup. **(a)** Using a concealer brush, I applied a very small amount of highlighting (light) concealer just to add some light: ● Underneath the eyes **(b)** Using an airbrush, I applied a pinky-beige foundation all over her face and neck.

2 Lips

Elizabeth called her lips "less than voluptuous." This is not surprising, since our lips naturally lose collagen and color as we age. Now listen up, ladies. Don't try to compensate for thinner lips by applying a darker colored lipstick to make your lips stand out. Applying dark lipstick actually has the effect of making your lips look smaller and creates what I like to call "zipper lips"—lips that look more like a zipper than they do lips. You don't want zipper lips. *Remember: Light adds and dark diminishes. If you want to enhance something, make it lighter. If you want to minimize something, make it darker.* **(a)** I applied a fleshy-beige lip liner with some pink in it to Elizabeth's lips. I wanted a little color to avoid having a completely nude lip; otherwise, Elizabeth's mouth would disappear completely. **(b)** I finished off with a pale pink lip gloss similar in color to the lip liner. The softness of the lip gloss creates a softer mouth as opposed to using lipstick, which tends to cake more easily.

(continued from page 117)

My mother used to say, "Just grow old gracefully." What she meant is that we should accept it and not fight it. I think differently. I don't mind getting older, but I don't want to look it, feel it, or act it. I take really good care of my skin, eat healthy food, and exercise. I keep myself active, both in body and in mind. I stay open to new ideas and keep current with the trends. Getting older has given me a kind of freedom. I am much more comfortable in my skin.

SCOTT: Do you think our society regards older women as beautiful, or are we a youth-obsessed society?

ELIZABETH: Yes, I think that some people think older women are beautiful. Meryl Streep, Katherine Hepburn, Sophia Loren—they exude a timeless beauty and have always presented themselves in a positive, confident, and classy way. Unfortunately, I also think we are a youth-obsessed society, which is sad because some of the youthful beauties that are emulated do not have the substance to be role models for today's youth.

SCOTT: How would your daughters describe you?

(continued on page 121)

Tip Remember, your face and neck should know each other. So blend your foundation down past your jawline or else you'll end up with the dreaded makeup line between the face and the neck.

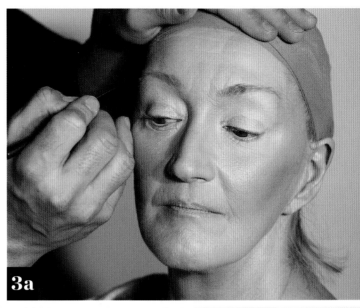

3a

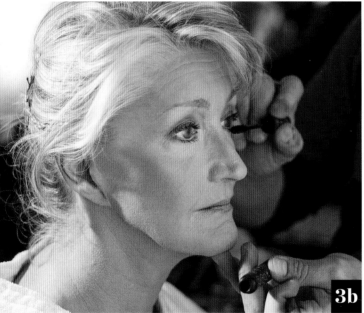

3b

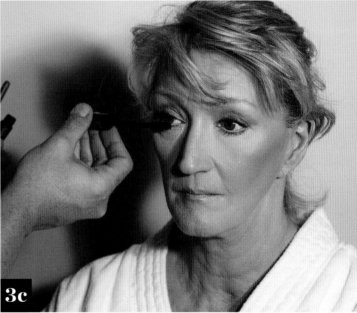

3c

Tip Heavy eyelashes on a mature woman make her look like an aging theatre star. So, use lighter lashes, unless, of course, you're going for really high drama!

(continued from page 119)

3 Eyes

With Elizabeth, I didn't want to create any kind of "look" where she would appear heavily made up, so I went with subtler shading. **(a)** I applied a subtle eye shadow called Cashmere (a pale brown-gray) in her crease to create hollows in the eye. **(b)** I applied white eyeliner on the inside of her lower eyelid instead of black eyeliner to help open up her eye. Black eyeliner would look too heavy with Elizabeth's fair coloring. **(c)** I added false eyelashes to give her eyes more oomph, but I used a strip in which the lashes were sparse and open. **(d)** I finished off the eyes with lots of black mascara on both the upper and lower lashes.

4 Eyebrows

Elizabeth doesn't have eyebrows due to years of over-plucking, so I created Elizabeth's eyebrows using an eyebrow pencil. Because of her lighter coloring, I didn't want to go too heavy on her brow. I used a very pale brown eyebrow pencil (almost a camel color) and followed her brow bone. This color provides a much warmer look than an icy gray pencil.

Remember: Always opt to use a razor comb for shaping your brows instead of plucking the hairs away. Plucking damages the follicles and eventually the follicles die. Your eyebrows require a bit more maintenance with a razor, but they still look nicely manicured without suffering permanent damage.

5 Blush

Elizabeth has terrific cheekbones, so I applied a soft peach cream blush, blending in a circular motion and making sure to stay on the apples of her cheeks. I wanted to use a subtle tone so that her face wouldn't scream, "Hey, I'm wearing blush!" With blush, when in doubt always go subtler; otherwise, you risk looking like Baby Jane Hudson or like you applied your makeup in the dark.

6 Setting the look

I finished off with a nice dusting of translucent powder so as not to change the color of the foundation and the blush.

Tip Applying blush on the apples of the cheeks makes the face more youthful; applying blush under the cheekbones slims the face and makes it appear drawn.

ELIZABETH: They say I'm a cool and hip mom. They all seem to value my opinions and ask for advice on things all the time because they know I will offer my opinion without being judgmental. Even though I am first and foremost a mom, my girls are also my friends.

SCOTT: You stay very active. How do you keep up your energy?
ELIZABETH: I am a very energetic person by nature. I get up early, exercise, and begin my day. I always look at a new day as being an opportunity to begin another adventure and to discover something new. My trick is working with youngsters. I teach horseback riding to 4-H kids. I also substitute teach. Kids keep you thinking young. My grandson does that every day.

SCOTT: Do you normally wear a lot of makeup?
ELIZABETH: It depends on what I've got going on. For my usual routine, I use mineral veil for powder, put on a little blush, some eye makeup, and that's about it. It takes me about twenty minutes. I take a little longer to do my hair, because I use hot curlers.

(continued on page 122)

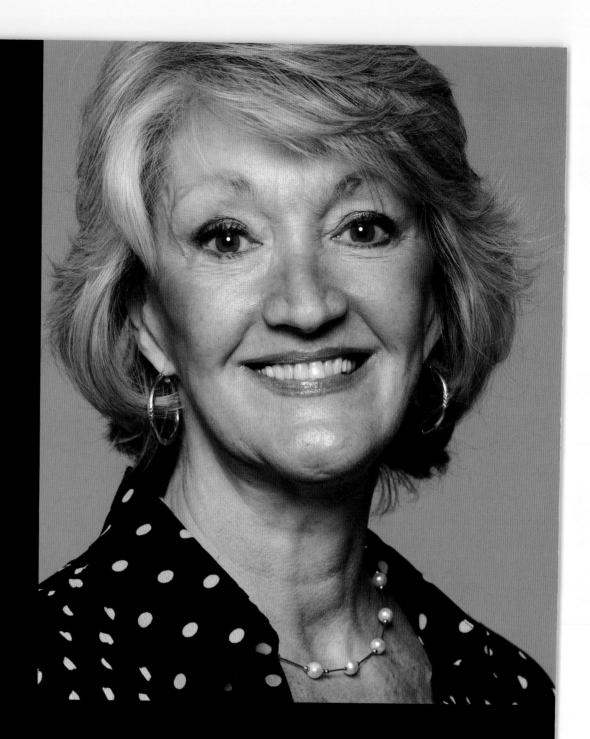

Elizabeth's Reaction
to Her Transformation

"Going into the day, I was very nervous because I thought, 'Oh my God, everyone's going to think I'm decrepit.' But everybody turned out to be so nice. I felt great about everything."

"I'm amazed at how Scott made me look. My first reaction was, 'I never thought I could look like this.' Looking at myself in the mirror, I felt extremely confident. The new hairstyle and the eyebrows—it's just amazing how those things make such a

(continued from page 121)

SCOTT: You have great skin. Do you do a lot for skin care?
ELIZABETH: I try to take care of my skin, yes. In the mornings when I take my shower, I scrub my face with one of those exfoliant cleansers, and then I put on my creams. I have three or four favorite creams I use and rotate: one with Retinol-A, one with DMAE (dimethylaminoethanol), one with peptides, and one with Alpha Hydroxy. In the evening, I do basically the same thing, but I use a heavier night cream.

SCOTT: When do you feel most confident?
ELIZABETH: I don't consider myself an overly confident person to begin with, but I think I feel best when I'm interacting with other people, making them laugh—when we're all enjoying ourselves. And on those days when my hair comes out good, which is rare!

difference. And making the eyes larger—I always thought I knew how to use makeup to enhance my eyes, but Scott taught me tricks that work even better. It just goes to show you can teach an old dog new tricks!"

"If I could describe myself before the makeover, it would probably be Elizabeth, the Sunday school teacher. But now I'd describe myself as Elizabeth, the sexy siren of the senior set!"

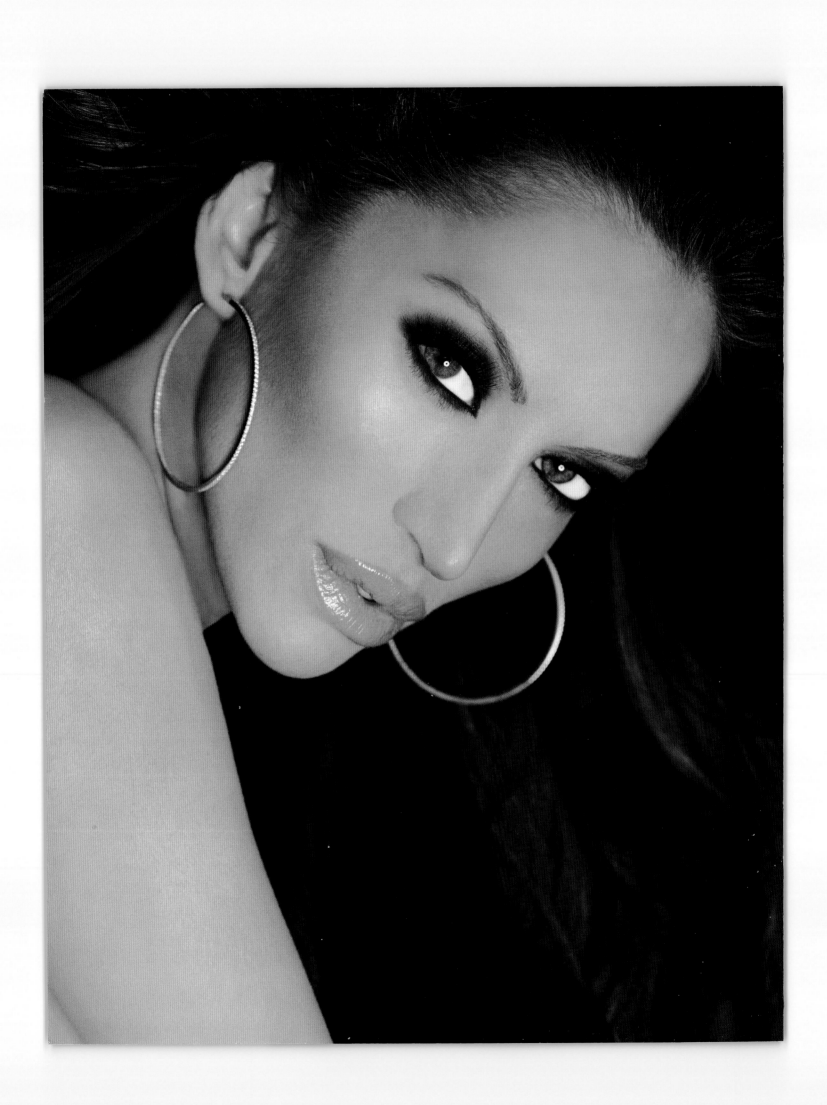

Evis:
Going Dramatic with Softer Colors

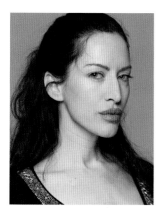

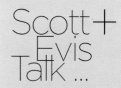

E vis has been one of my closest friends for years. She was born and raised in Albania, but she's now a film and television actress who has lived in Los Angeles for the past eight years. Evis also dates a rock star and could easily live the life of a wild child consisting of drinking, drugs, and frivolity that the industry is famous for. But she doesn't. She's disciplined, she has strong values, and she makes it a point to stay grounded.

In her life, as in her acting, Evis is fearless. That includes not being afraid to experiment with her appearance. In fact, I never quite know what she'll look like the next time I see her because she's always changing her hair color. The day of her makeover, Evis came in with very dark hair and pink lips that, although dramatic, were too severe for her coloring and minimized her best features. I decided to warm up and balance her look. Now, instead of one feature, we focus in on a strikingly beautiful woman.

SCOTT: I see you've changed your hair color again.
EVIS: You know me; I like to change it every six months, depending on my mood. People treat you differently depending on your hair color. There really is that thing that when you're blonde, guys think you're a little ditzy. But they take you more seriously with dark hair. I had red hair for a period of time, too.

SCOTT: I remember. Is there anything else besides your hair color that you would like to change about yourself?
EVIS: I'm not sure what I would change about myself. I'm kind of used to my face by now. If we're talking about other parts of the body? I'd say better boobs-subtle, not too big [laughs]. Is there a makeup to help with that?

SCOTT: If you could figure that out, you'd make lots of money! Let's talk about your beauty regimen. What do you do on a regular basis?
EVIS: In the morning I wash my face with cold water and then apply moisturizer and

(continued on page 127)

Creating Evis's Look

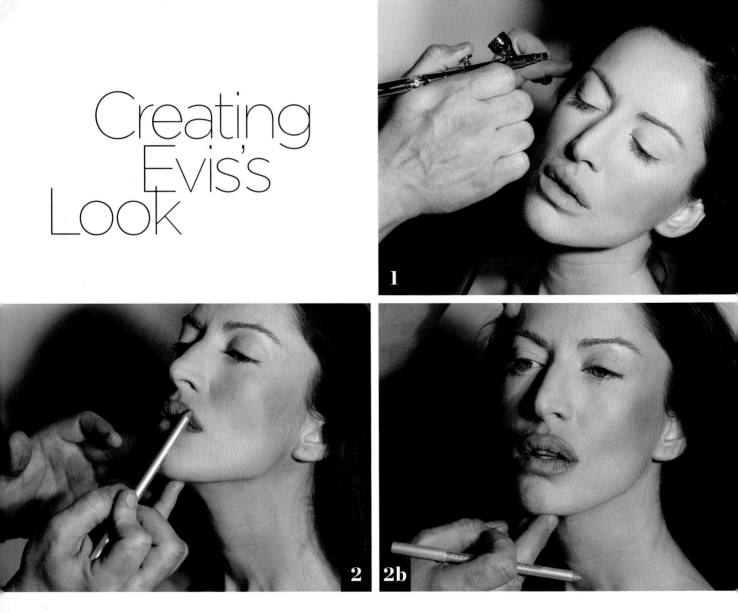

Tip You can line your lips in one of two places:
• Just inside the lip line to soften fuller lips • Right
on the border of the lip for normal to smaller lips
I never recommend lining outside the border of the
lip. Read that last statement again. I have a name
for the look this kind of lining creates, but it's not
appropriate to put in print, so I'll just call it clown
mouth. Stay away from lining outside the lip.
Stay away from clown mouth.

(continued from page 125)

Evis likes a dramatic look, so she tends to go for sharp contrasts in coloring. I wanted to show her how she could still create high drama with softer, warmer colors that draw out her own features, particularly her fantastic eyes.

....

1 Contouring, highlighting, and foundation

Evis doesn't like a lot of foundation, but I still wanted to warm up the color of her skin without it feeling like too much makeup. As I did for Elizabeth, I chose to airbrush Evis's foundation, which in Evis's case would provide even coverage without feeling like heavy makeup.

With an airbrush, I applied a light beige foundation with a warm tone all over her face and neck. Evis has very pale skin, so I didn't want to go too dark with her foundation. Just adding this tiny bit of color significantly warmed up her overall coloring. I used no highlighter or concealer on Evis. Instead, I let the lighter airbrush foundation suffice for the highlight.

2 Lips

Evis has really full, really beautiful lips, but the last thing I wanted to do was overemphasize them with lip lining, especially because I wanted to switch the focus from her lips to her extraordinary greenish-blue eyes. However, I still want to give the lips some definition. **(a)** Using a flesh-colored lip liner, I lined just slightly inside the border of her lips. A color any darker would have drawn more focus toward her lips, which I didn't want to do. **(b)** I finished off the lips with a peachy-colored gloss.

an eye cream. And then at night I usually do a face scrub with an exfoliator. My skin is combination skin. I also exercise—not a lot, but a little bit of yoga and a little bit of cardio.

SCOTT: What else do you do to stay beautiful?
EVIS: Probably the biggest thing I do that makes a difference is I drink nothing but water, smoothies and juices—no soda, no coffee, and no alcohol. It's the best thing for my skin and body. And I stay out of the sun.

SCOTT: Do you follow a special diet, too?
EVIS: I eat pretty healthy, pretty much everything organic, including organic meat with no hormones. I eat vegetables, a lot of sushi, and I drink lots of water. My boyfriend says I eat a lot, so I think I have a very high metabolism.

SCOTT: You travel a lot. Is there anything you do differently for your skin when traveling?
EVIS: Yes, I apply extra moisturizer. And I don't usually wear foundation when I travel, because I like to let my skin breathe. I also drink a lot more water.

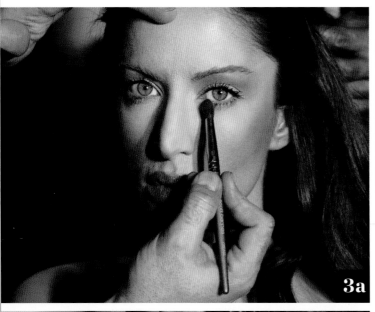

3a

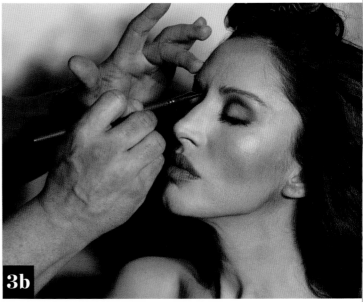

3b

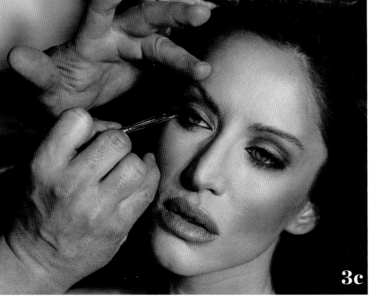

3c

Tip Using a warmer eye shadow for the base is a good idea if you also intend to use darker colors to create a "smoky" look. The warmer color helps soften the look overall by blending the line between the darker and lighter sections of the eye.

3 Eyes

Evis has very pale greenish-blue eyes that are stunning—they deserve emphasis. When applying the eye shadow, I used different eye shadow brushes for each step for cleaner application. Using separate brushes is the best way to avoid mixing eye shadow colors in their cases. **(a)** Using a tapered eye shadow brush, I surrounded the eye with gold leaf eye shadow—putting it on the lid, in the crease, and under the eye—before laying in the darker colors. The purpose of this was not only to create warmth and bring out the blue in her eyes but also to unify the canvas, which allowed me to build up from there. **(b)** I then layered burgundy eye shadow over the gold eye shadow in the crease of the eye to create more dimension. **(c)** I also put this burgundy eye color underneath the eye and in the outer corners. The reddish tone helped draw out the blue in Evis's pupils. **(d)** I used a brown Maybelline pencil to line inside of her upper and lower eyelids. **(e)** I completed the eye with some medium-density false eyelashes.

4 Cheeks

I wanted to go with very subtle blush on Evis's cheeks to keep the focus drawn toward her eyes. So, I used natural colors that simply warmed up her face without adding a lot of color. **(a)** Moving the blush brush in a circular motion, I applied a cream peach-colored blush to the apples of her cheeks. **(b)** With a separate bronzing brush, I lightly dusted loose bronzing powder on top of the blush to bring more warmth into the peachy tone. **(c)** I delicately applied a small amount of champagne shimmer highlight on top of the cheekbones.

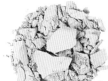

Tip With shimmer highlight, a little bit goes a very long way for reflecting the light. So, be careful not to spill excess powder on other parts of your cheeks or face.

REACTIONS...

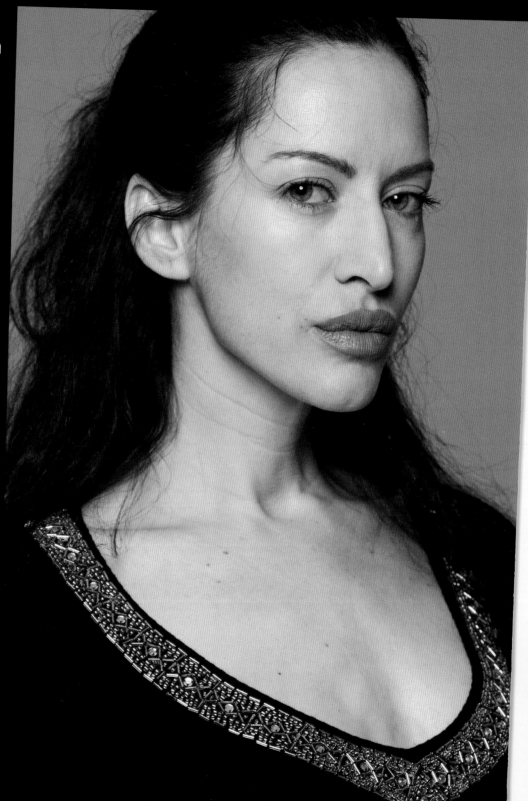

Evis's Reaction to Her Transformation

"Scott is not just another makeup artist; he's a real force of nature. I mean, look at the difference in me! He can transform a woman from regular to extraordinary. I've worked with Scott a few other times and I'm always impressed with how meticulous he is. The way he works is very, very thorough. But it's not just because of the way he applies the makeup. Scott also has a way of stripping away a person's insecurities during the process. That's a fierce makeover. I'm also excited about trying some of these new colors. Looking like I have a warmer skin tone changes me completely. And the reddish-browns he used definitely make my eyes stand out more; like they're a brighter bluish-green. Once again, Scott has taught me something new. I'm lucky to have a friend who's such a master of beauty."

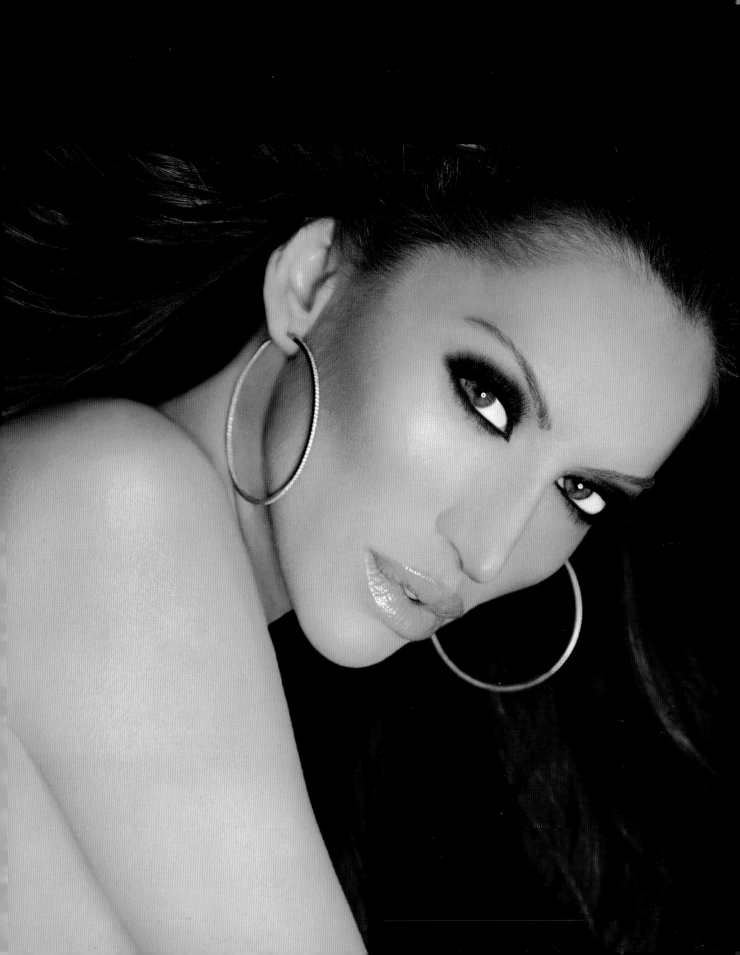

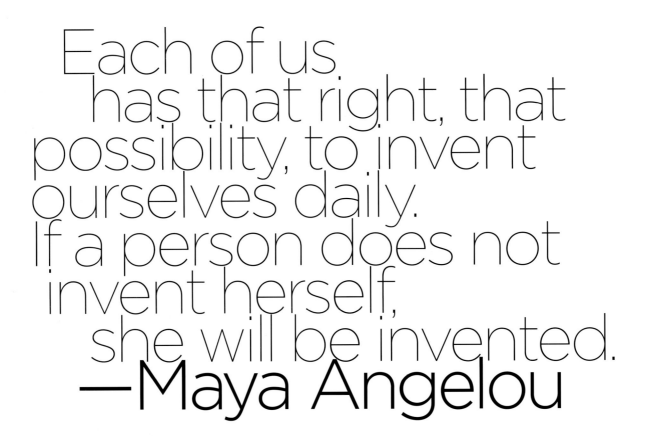

Each of us
    has that right, that
possibility, to invent
ourselves daily.
If a person does not
invent herself,
    she will be invented.
    —Maya Angelou

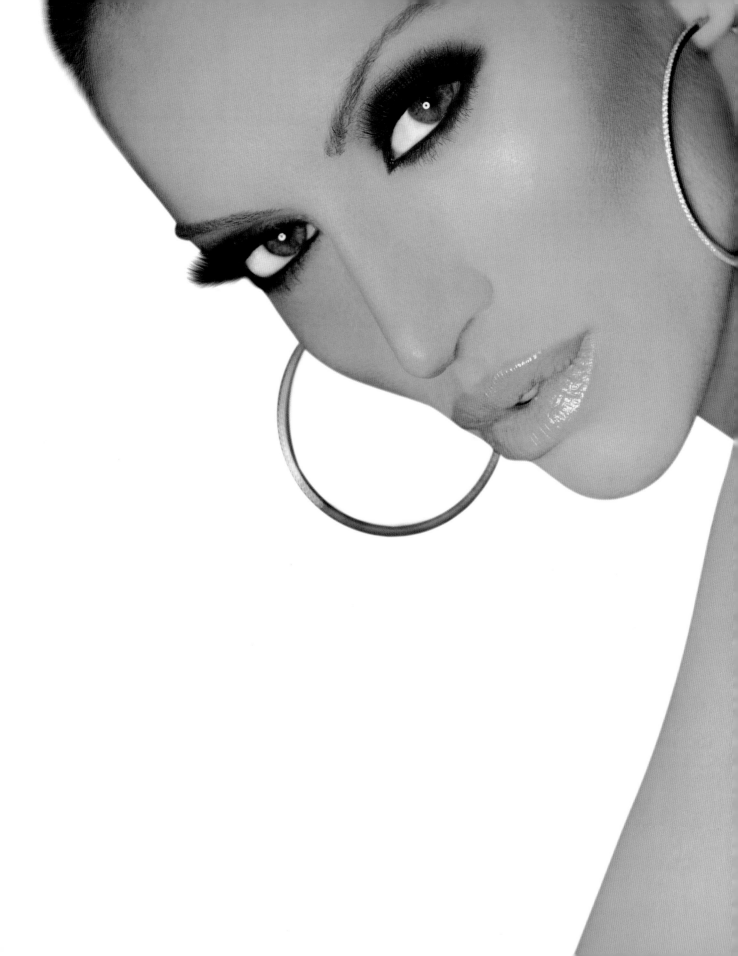

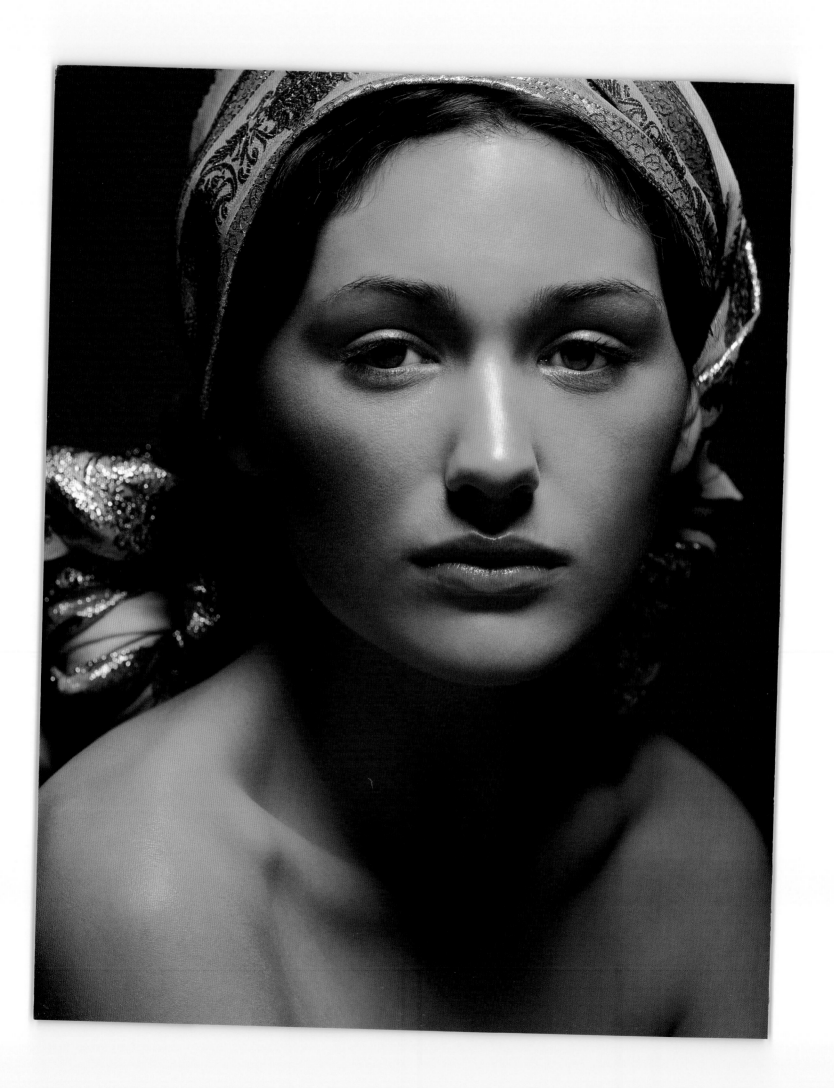

Sarah:
Applying Makeup for Natural, No-Makeup Beauty

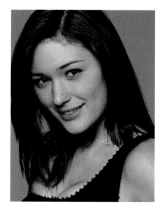

Makeup doesn't always have to be about changing your look or creating drama. Sometimes less is definitely more. Sarah's face—with her French–Italian features and coloring—conjures up portraits from the neoclassical period. Her flawless skin gives her the option of using makeup to merely enhance her beauty for a natural, no-makeup look. But this kind of minimal look isn't achieved by simply walking out the door without makeup. Creating the illusion of "fresh and naturally beautiful" still requires a little time and effort. But as Sarah's transformation reveals, it can definitely be worth it. This look is just as relevant today as it was centuries ago.

SCOTT: How do you keep your skin looking so good?
SARAH: I've been lucky in that I've never really had skin problems. So, I've never had to do anything special. I wash my face in the morning and at night. Anything more than that, especially in New York weather, is too much. It dries my skin out like crazy. I wash my face with Murad Clarifying Cleanser, and then I put on a moisturizer right after. I just started moisturizing about a year ago, when I should've been doing it all along, but that has really, really changed my skin. Now that I moisturize in the morning and at night, I hardly ever break out.

SCOTT: Do you have to stick to a special diet to maintain your good skin?
SARAH: Well, I don't eat fried food. I love popcorn, but I also try to stay away from salty foods. I eat a lot of protein, like grilled fish and grilled chicken, and steamed vegetables. In the morning, I'll eat some fruit or some oatmeal. I drink coffee. But mostly I drink water. I recently stopped drinking

(continued on page 137)

Creating Sarah's Look

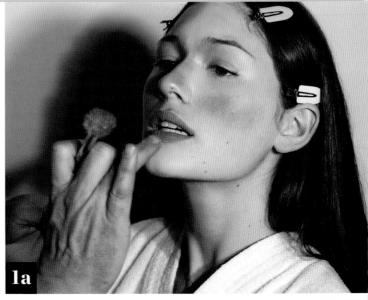

1a

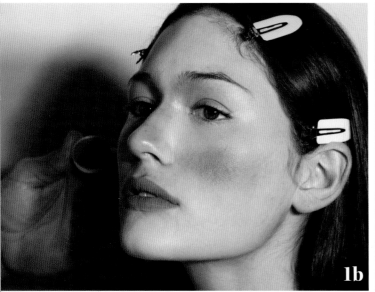

1b

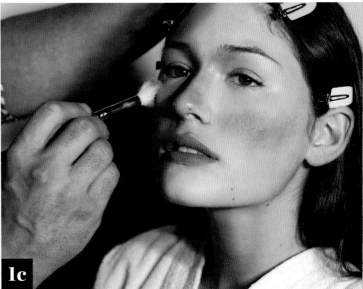

1c

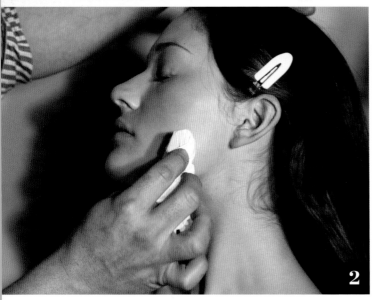

2

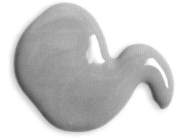

The better your skin is, the more likely you'll be able to pull off the no-makeup look since it's really about taking healthy skin and making it look healthier. So, first make sure your skin is in the best possible shape—hydrated, with no significant marks or blemishes. (See "The Skinny on Skin" chapter for ways to maintain healthy skin.)

Instead of powder, I used oils and shimmers to highlight the top of Sarah's cheekbones and the end of her nose. This look isn't about using a lot of color. In fact, I achieved this whole look using only three colors: wine-burgundy, champagne, and gold. I recommend using only berry and wine colors for this look, as they are the same colors found in nature.

1 Contouring, highlighting, and foundation

Sarah already has healthy, glowing skin, so I used cream-based products for her contouring, highlighting, and foundation. **(a)** Using a goat hair brush, I applied contouring (dark) foundation: ● Underneath the cheekbones ● On the sides of the nose ● At the inner eye where the bridge of the nose meets the brow bone ● At the temples **(b)** Using a concealer brush, I brought out all her bones using highlights and shimmery creams. I applied the highlighting (light) concealer: ● Underneath the eyes ● On top of the cheekbones ● Underneath the eyebrows ● On the bridge of the nose ● At the center of the chin ● In the center of the forehead **(c)** Using a separate goat hair brush, I applied a foundation that matched her skin coloring on top of the contouring and highlighting. I blended in a circular motion with a very light touch for a flawless finish.

2 Setting the look

Before adding translucent powder, I wanted to absorb any excess makeup and push it into the skin so that it blended with her natural oils. **(a)** I placed a makeup sponge in the center of a tissue. I then twisted the tissue around the sponge, as though I were wrapping a Hershey's kiss. **(b)** I lightly dabbed the tissue-sponge onto her skin. **(c)** I then applied a light dusting of translucent powder in the T-zone (chin, bridge of the nose, forehead, and underneath the eyes) to remove excess shine.

For the rest of the process I used nothing but cream-based makeup, which is very close to the consistency of lipstick. In fact, I've been known to achieve a very similar look with nothing but one tube of lipstick!

(continued from page 135)

as much alcohol as I used to. On the weekends, I'll go out and have a drink, but otherwise, hardly ever. I also drink a Diet Coke from time to time. My dad is an orthodontist, so growing up it was always "no soft drinks in the house, it's so bad for your teeth." So, we'd have to sneak them!

SCOTT: And how about exercise?
SARAH: I've been getting into Pilates and yoga two or three times a week. And I jog.

SCOTT: Do you like to wear a lot of makeup?
SARAH: I like to experiment when I go out, so I'll do smoky eyes or some crazy colors but still try to be fairly natural with it. I have roommates who take hours to get ready, but they are so naturally beautiful already. I don't understand why they need to do all the things they do to themselves.

SCOTT: How would you describe your everyday fashion style?

(continued on page 139)

An important part of the
NO-MAKEUP, RADIANT SKIN LOOK
is creating healthy
flush colored cheeks.

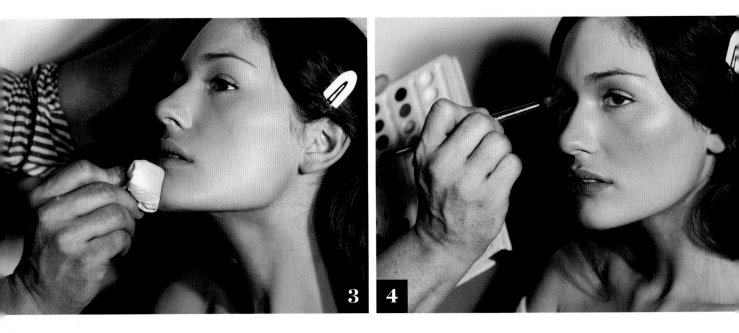

Tip When searching for a cream highlighter for your cheekbones, look for shimmery champagne colors, if you're Caucasian. If you're dark-skinned, the highlighter should have a warm, copper tone to it.

Tip Use a light touch during application. Again, you want the look of minimal makeup.

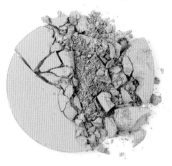

3 Cheeks

An important part of the no-makeup, radiant skin look is creating healthy, flush colored cheeks. **(a)** Using my fingers, I applied to the apples of her cheeks a wine-colored cream blush that was the same color I would be using on her lips. **(b)** Using a blush brush, I blended this color into the shimmery highlight cream, so there would be no separation between these two colors.

4 Eyes

For Sarah's eyes, I simply wanted to add a small bit of color to her lids for a bit of dimension. **(a)** I put a gold cream across the whole lid. **(b)** I then applied champagne-colored highlighter just under the brow bone. I put no mascara on Sarah; however, if you want mascara with this kind of minimal look, here's what I recommend: **(a)** Curl your lashes with your eyelash curler. **(b)** Wipe most of the mascara off the wand with a tissue, so there's a minimal amount on the brush. **(c)** Rub the end of the mascara wand with the tips of your index finger and thumb to stain them with some color. *Note: Clean fingers will ensure you don't get any bacteria on the wand.* **(d)** Apply the mascara on your lashes using your fingers, instead of the mascara brush. This will give a "tint" of color on the lashes, without looking like you've applied mascara.

5 Lips

The trick to creating lips that look like they're naturally flushed is to use a stain that's slightly darker than your natural lip color. This gives the impression that the lips are flush and healthy. You don't want to use any kind of gloss or frosted color that looks artificial or heavily covers the lip. **(a)** I first wanted to get the blood flowing to Sarah's lips. So, with a small, natural-bristle brush I brushed some lip balm lightly, back and forth, on both the top and bottom lips. This helps plump the lips as well as gets rid of any dead skin. **(b)** With my finger, I then applied the same cream cheek-colored stain on Sarah's lips that I used on the apples of her cheeks.

(continued from page 137)

SARAH: I wear a lot of my boyfriend's clothes—so, boyish and edgy.

SCOTT: What do you like to do outside of modeling?
SARAH: I love to read and write. I read all sorts of different things. And I write a lot. I eventually plan on going back to school for creative writing. I wrote for my hometown newspaper in Mississippi when I was in seventh and eigth grade. So ever since then, I've always wanted to write for magazines about beauty and skin care.

SCOTT: Do you have any kind of life philosophy?
SARAH: I feel that whatever good, positive energy you put out into the world, that's what will come back to you. And I think it helps to be open to things and for making new friends all the time. What's the point of being negative?

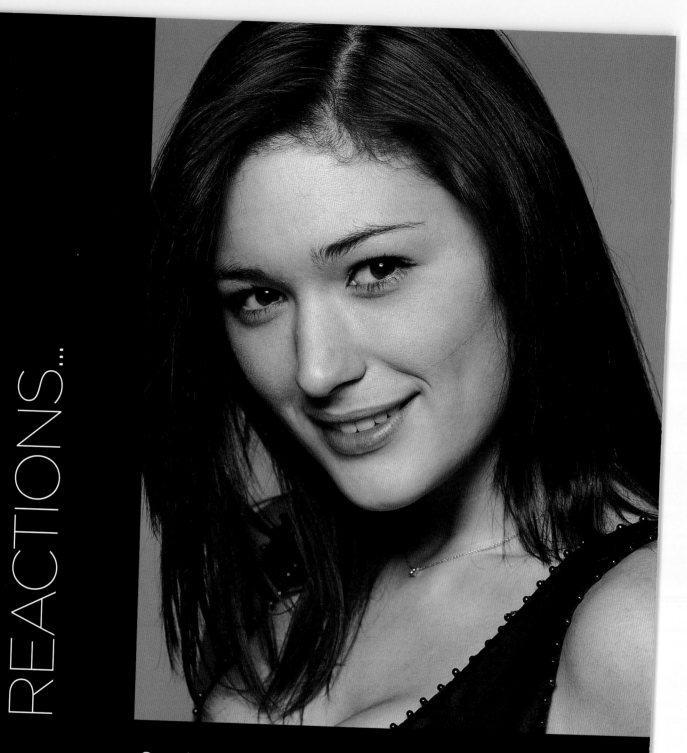

REACTIONS...

Sarah's Reaction to Her Transformation

"The result was beautiful. Scott made my skin literally glow. It was funny, because I told him in the beginning that I loved the natural look the best, and generally that I like to keep that the goal when doing my own makeup. So, I was so excited to see how he would do the no-makeup look. He didn't even use mascara. That's about as natural as it gets!"

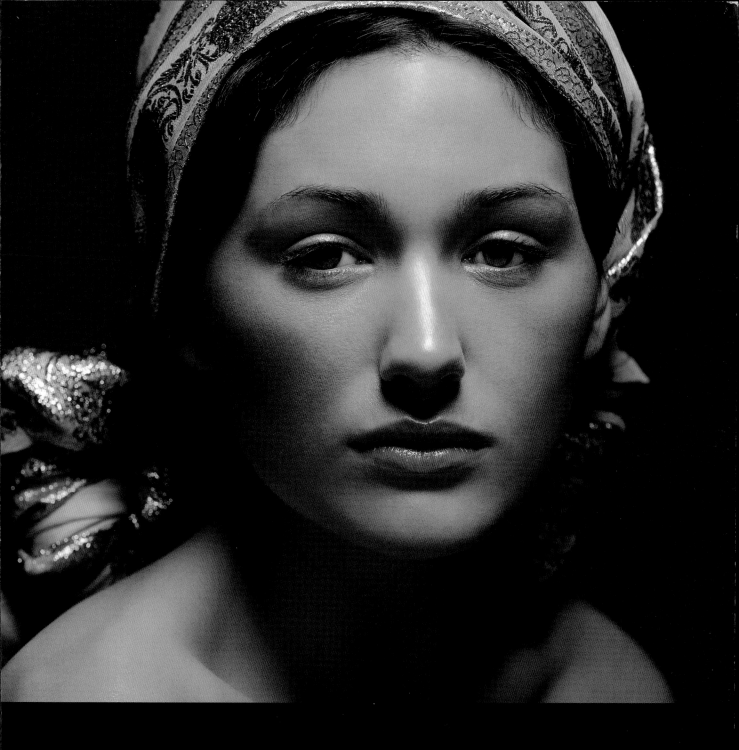

"Before Scott, I would use a little bit of eyeliner on my top lids only, but since he showed me how I can make my skin look better while using less makeup, I realized that using dark eyeliner was actually making my face look older in a way. So, I definitely don't do that anymore. I really feel the new techniques give me a fresher, younger look."

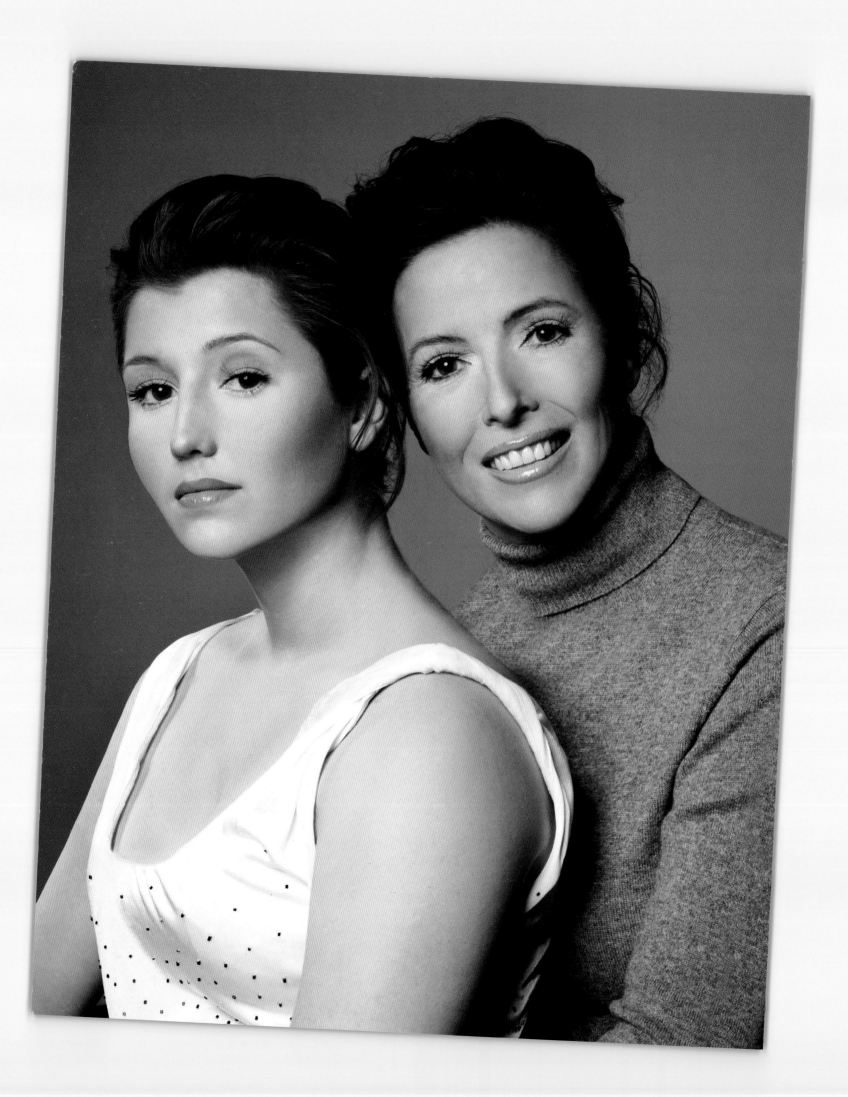

The Skinny on Skin

In many ways, this chapter on skin should precede all the others, because there's really nothing more important than healthy, radiant skin when it comes to beauty. It's the canvas on which a look is created. Having bad skin is like starting with a canvas that's torn or stained—you spend your whole time working around and covering blemishes. Fortunately, today it's easier than it used to be to have great skin. And that's what this chapter is about: how to give your skin some loving so that it glows.

People often wonder why they don't look as good as many celebrities. They attribute a star's good looks to something they can't personally achieve themselves. I hear it all the time: "Star X must have been born with good genes" or "The gods blessed Star Y when they made her." Well, here's the inside scoop: These so-called natural beauties work at it. Their beauty, in large part, is due to how they take care of their bodies. They make sure to exercise on a regular basis, they make healthy food choices, and they put long-term gain ahead of short-term gratification. And when they indulge every now and then—which they do because they're only human—they do what it takes to make up for it.

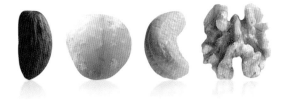

Another thing you can do for your skin is GET PLENTY OF PROTEIN. —Dr. Eva

Antioxidants exist as vitamins (namely A, C and E), enzymes, and other compounds in foods.

Scott: It's a pretty simple equation: what you put in your body gets reflected on how you look on the outside.

Dr. Eva: That's a great way to put it. Another thing you can do for your skin is get plenty of protein. Protein is the natural building block for healthy collagen, and as we all know, collagen keeps your skin firm and toned...kind of like a yoga class for your skin!

Scott: Firm and tone with protein, ladies!

Dr. Eva: One last, very important thing I would like to mention: Provide some TLC with EFAs. Essential fatty acids (EFAs) are as essential to your diet as vitamins. They provide tender, loving care for your skin as well as your arteries and heart. They're even great for relieving PMS and monthly breast pain. EFAs cannot be produced in from within our body, so we must include them in our diet. There are two important families of EFAs: Omega 6s found in plant oils, nuts, seeds, and soybeans and Omega 3s found in cold water fish, cod liver oil, and flax seed.

Omega 6s can also be taken in the form of supplements. Just be sure to look for Omega 6 supplements that have been purified and are mercury-free. There are many cheap non-purified Omega 6 supplements out there which can lead to mercury toxicity.

So whether you enjoy a handful of nuts, a nice fish dinner, or take your Omega 6s in the form of supplements, just make sure you regularly lubricate your skin with EFAs.

Scott: We all know a little lubrication can go a very long way...Thank you, Dr. Eva!

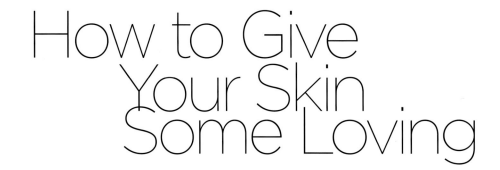

How to Give Your Skin Some Loving

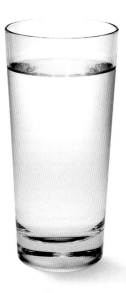

the fake tan? Too much exposure to the sun makes you look like an old Gucci bag. Unsexy! This is why I created Body Bling and other self tanners, so you can get a gorgeous tan without risking overexposure to those nasty UVA rays.

Restore with Sleep

They call it "beauty sleep" for a reason. Sleep and beauty really are interrelated. Everything regenerates when you sleep. Your mind renews, your cells renew, and your skin renews. I like to believe that when I'm sleeping, a housekeeper comes in and tidies up, making the bed and ironing out my wrinkles and removing the toxins from the night before. She restores the whole house before I have to get up and at it the next morning.

Body builders also understand the importance of restorative sleep. Their first rule of thumb is to get plenty of sleep after a hard workout. They know they won't see any improvement in their muscles until they've slept and given their muscles time to rebuild. So, never feel guilty about sneaking a nap or sleeping in. If you feel tired, it's your body telling you it needs time

to repair. You'll be rewarded with healthier skin when you wake up!

Shed the Dead (Skin)

It's important to exfoliate twice a month to remove the dead cells on the top layer of your skin. Dead skin is the chief reason for skin appearing dull and dry, so when you exfoliate, you immediately gain a more youthful luster to your skin. The increased blood flow that results from invigorated skin also helps stimulate collagen growth. Dead skin also tends to block pores and trap bacteria, so regular exfoliation can also help control acne. But remember: Do not exfoliate more than twice a month. Overexfoliation can be damaging to your skin; if you begin to strip away healthy cells in addition to the dead cells, this can lead to an outbreak of acne. The best indication that you're overexfoliating is if your skin feels irritated or you see increased redness. Your skin should be pleasantly tingly, not burning , after exfoliating.

Create Your Own Tropical Paradise

You don't have to go to the tropics to achieve the benefits that humidity and moisture provide to your skin. You can create your own tropical paradise with a humidifier and a few plants. Or you can invest in a miniature fountain, which is a more aesthetically pleasing humidifier. Whatever you buy, the point is to moisten the air with H_2O. This is particularly important in the winter when the dry air from heaters sucks the moisture from your skin. Also, did you know that your skin dehydrates when your sleep? And dehydration causes skin to wrinkle and sag. See where I'm going with this? So, if you don't want to run your humidifier all the time, use it only at night. Placing some plants around is also nice, not only because they liven up your surroundings (quite literally) but also because research has shown that plants help you feel more relaxed and prompt you to breathe deeper, allowing more oxygen to enter your system. Plants also help to remove chemicals—toxins—from the air.

Indulge in a Night of Beauty

I'm all about pampering with facials, massages, and whatnot. But I don't believe it has to cost a mint. Give yourself a break both physically and financially by staying home one night a month to indulge in a "night of beauty." Luxuriate in a hot bath filled with body oils while drinking a seltzer with mint. Give yourself a home facial. Have some good sex or fantasize about good sex. It's all about letting go of the tension and thoroughly relaxing so that you breathe deep and easy. The increased oxygen in your blood is a wonderful boost for your skin.

The best news is that our skin cells are constantly regenerating. So if you have problem skin or you've damaged your skin, there are many, many things you can do, starting today, to have better skin. You can minimize skin damage or get rid of it altogether, thanks to technological advances in skin care, whether they be creams, injections or more advanced treatments.

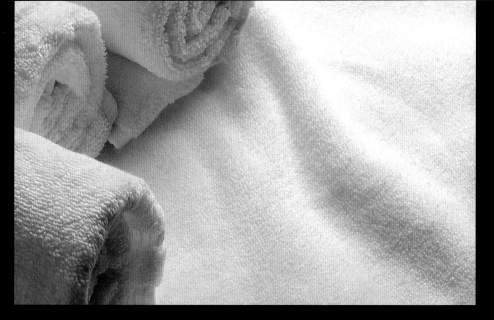

Home Facial Recipe

To give yourself a facial, follow these steps: **(1)** Put on some relaxing music. **(2)** Boil some water in a covered quart-size pot, with or without chamomile herbs. **(3)** While you're waiting for the water to boil, cleanse your face and then grab a very large towel or blanket. **(4)** When the water comes to a boil, remove the pot from the stove and place it somewhere where you can sit comfortably with your face leaning over it. (You can also stand at the stove, but it's less comfortable.) **(5)** Remove the lid and let some of the initial steam escape before putting your face into the steam. **(6)** Cover your head and the pot with the blanket or towel. **(7)** Sit in your tent of steam and breathe deeply for seven to ten minutes. **(8)** Pat your face dry, apply a moisturizing mask, and leave it on for fifteen minutes. **(9)** Remove the mask with cool water. **(10)** Follow with a good moisturizer.
Voilà! You now have happier, suppler skin!

Skin Damage and How You Can Avoid It

My good friend Dr. Jessica Wu is considered one of the top skin doctors in the United States. Recently, I sat down with Dr. Wu—along with Maureen Kornowa and her daughter, Marley, whom I had met at the annual Make a Wish Charity—to discuss the importance of caring for your skin.

SCOTT: How does a person know when to seek out a skin specialist?

DR. WU: As soon as something starts to bother you, then you should visit a doctor. That's not to say some people aren't deluded sometimes. I've had sixteen- and seventeen-year-olds who believe they have a frown line and come in for a Botox injection. I send them home. But the general rule of thumb is, when something starts to bother you, it's time to see a dermatologist. And you may not need an injection or laser; you may simply need a topical Retin-A cream or a topical antioxidant. But there are definitely things we can do to help improve what you have as well as prevent further lines from appearing.

SCOTT: So, since everyone can't fly to Los Angeles and get an appointment with the fabulous Dr. Wu, how does someone go about finding a top dermatologist?

DR. WU: One of the best places to start is with your regular doctor. Or you can usually get a good referral from your makeup artist or your facialist or even your hairstylist because these people are in the business of beauty and appearance. A lot of times, their clients will talk about a good or bad experience if they've had one, so they will know someone who has a reputation for doing good work.

SCOTT: In other words, don't pick your doctor out of the yellow pages and certainly not from one of those late night television commercials. How often do you recommend people see a dermatologist?

DR. WU: I strongly recommend people come in once a year, and in the course of doing a mole examination, we'll talk about other things. For example, people will notice a lot of sun damage on their cheeks that they want to clear up. Or they have acne concerns.

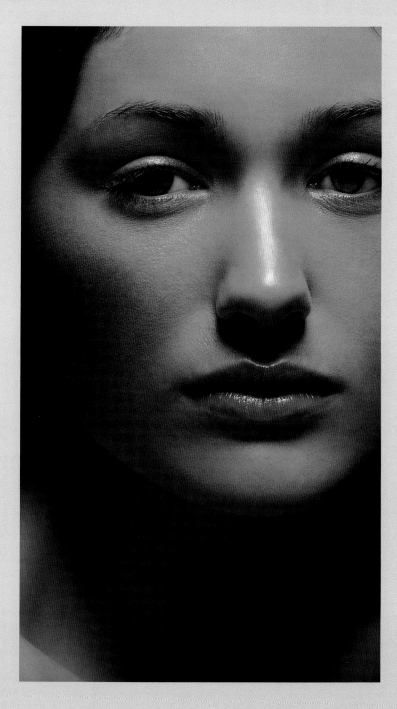

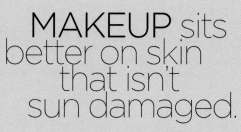

MAKEUP sits better on skin that isn't sun damaged.

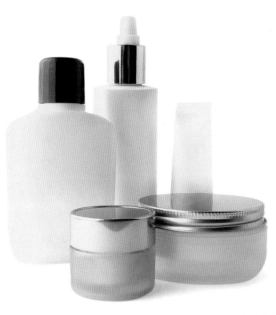

SCOTT: I think makeup sits better on skin that isn't sun damaged. The skin is easier to cover when you have an even skin tone and when you're skin's softer, more supple. The makeup looks more like it's a part of your skin, not like it's sitting on top.

DR. WU: Yes, I think your job is much easier when someone has good skin versus when someone comes in and they're all weather-beaten.

SCOTT: What are your thoughts about sun block?

DR. WU: I recommend using a lotion with an SPF of at least 30. And just as important as the SPF when looking for ingredients is that the product protects against UVA rays. UVAs are the aging rays. The SPF number only tells you how good the product is at protecting you from burning. When I was creating my skin-care line in the lab, the list of ingredients for SPF was overwhelming. I cut through all of those ingredients and realized that the three key ingredients for skin-care protection are zinc, titanium, or mexoryl, so make sure you're getting a product that includes at least one of these.

The other point I want to make is that a lot of my patients come in because their makeup artist notices a suspicious spot. These people are right there, up in their faces. Or their massage therapists or their facialists notice things. That's definitely the reason why it's good to have relationships with these other beauty professionals. So, listen when your makeup artist notices something or your hairstylist tells you there's something in your scalp. Listen to them.

SCOTT: That's true. People should check their scalp and between their toes. Doctors don't usually do that. And a lot of dermatologists don't check between the toes. I've never been to anybody but you, Jessica, who has checked between my toes.

DR. WU: It's a good idea to check everywhere for anything that wasn't there before.

SCOTT: Since we're talking about noticing things on your skin, we've got to address the issue of skin cancer. Skin care isn't just about beauty, it's also about protecting yourself and being smart about taking care of your skin, so you don't run the risk of getting skin

The three key ingredients for **SKIN-CARE PROTECTION** are zinc, titanium, *or mexoryl.*

cancer. And that's where Maureen and Marley come in. You look at their photo and you see two beautiful people who just seem to glow. But what you don't see is that Marley is a seventeen-year-old girl dealing with Stage 3 melanoma, the deadliest form of skin cancer. And this is something Marley and her mother and father have been dealing with over the past year.

MAUREEN: It's been a challenging year, to say the least.

SCOTT: Having lost my thirty-year-old brother to melanoma two years ago, I understand much of what you've been going through. Cancer moves in, and you've got a new member of the family, and you want them to leave already.

MARLEY: It's like a third person in the room.

MAUREEN: In the past year, we've been on a journey that began the day Marley received her diagnosis of Stage 3 cancer. Even though the journey had a lot of setbacks and detours in the beginning and some ugly news, Marley, in particular, hit that road on that journey with perseverance and laughter. We've found cancer humorous because it made the bad days a little bit easier. We thought, "Oh, if we're going to

sit here and go through this, we're going to have some fun doing it."

MARLEY: I named my pickline "Fiero" from the play Wicked, because Fiero was kind of sweet, and we put a scarf on it and I took Fiero to homecoming. We laugh at stuff like that.

SCOTT: You have to poke fun at it, because otherwise it starts beating you. It's good; it's healthy to play around with it.

MAUREEN: There are really two ways to approach life: Let it get you and curl up and die, or hold your head up high and laugh and do what's got to be done. With Marley, there was never any question which road it was going to be. From day one, she held her head high.

MARLEY: I believe there's a reason I have cancer. And part of the reason is cancer has brought my family closer. It has taught me things and taught us about being a family. I thank cancer for that.

SCOTT: And that's my attraction to you. You both possess such grace and dignity under such difficult circumstances. That personifies beauty for me. It's that inner strength and that inner beauty that just radiates, and it shows in your photograph. I saw it the day I met you. Out of all those people in the room, I was automatically drawn to you guys. And you don't run across that every day.

MAUREEN: Having gone through this experience with Marley's cancer, I would say that I have learned that you've got to get yourself checked once a year by a dermatologist, regardless of your age. I think there's a common misconception out there among the general populace that you shouldn't start getting your skin checked until you're older. But the truth is that melanoma is becoming more and more prevalent in younger people. You're not too young to have a deadly skin disease.

DR. WU: That's right. In general, everyone should get their skin checked once a year regardless of their age. Just like you get your blood pressure checked or your cholesterol checked or women do their mammograms or pelvic exams once a year, they should also get their skin checked. That's because skin cancer is one of the most preventable cancers. I tell patients, "If you can see it, then you can remove it early enough; it's curable." The problem comes up when people think that just because

it's on your skin and not internal, it's not really a problem. So, they ignore it. My response to that is, while it may not hurt you initially or you may not feel pain initially, if you wait too long it can travel internally and be potentially devastating.

So, the bottom line is everyone should get their skin checked once a year and even more frequently—every six months—if you have a history of skin cancer in your family, if the doctors ever found anything suspicious on you, and especially if you were sunburned as a child. We know that blistering sunburns and the use of tanning beds increase your risk. So, if you've had sunburns or used a tanning bed, you should start in your teens and twenties.

SCOTT: Tanning beds are shaped like a coffin for a reason.

DR. WU: So true.

SCOTT: And I'm guilty of being a tanner myself. But I've been educated through things like my brother's death and through not wanting to age. The work that you and I have done to reverse the damage has been enlightening, to say the least. Don't risk it by baking yourself!

MAUREEN: I want to point out that Marley is not someone who used

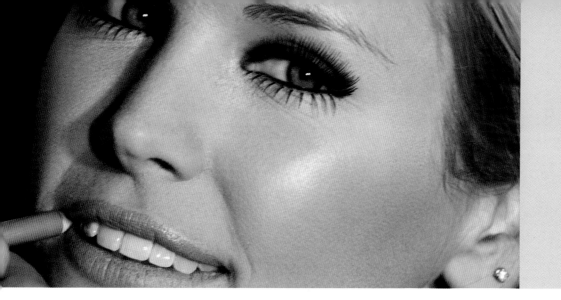

a tanning bed or who fried herself by laying out in the sun. She's an average, healthy teenager. Doctors now believe there may be a genetic connection, something hereditary. Although that wasn't even the case in our family—no one else in our families had ever had cancer. So, have your young kids checked once a year, period.

SCOTT: When faced with such a difficult, all-consuming challenge, the question becomes, how are you going to deal with it? In spite of your condition, Marley, you are still a beautiful young woman with a positive attitude and enough courage not only to get up and speak in front of hundreds of people, but to speak about something as personal as your cancer.

MARLEY: Thanks. I just believe it's what I'm supposed to do.

SCOTT: Well, you're a real inspiration to all of us.

MAUREEN: You can see why I'm so proud. And she always makes the point when she speaks: Don't underestimate skin cancer.

DR. WU: That's right, which is why it's important to do your own self-examinations every now and then.

SCOTT: What should people look for?

DR. WU: Look for any kind of change. That's why it's important to check your skin yourself once a month because as your doctor whom you see only once a year I'm not going to know what's changing. My job is to give you a baseline when you come in once a year, and your job is once a month or so to take a look at yourself and see if there are any changes. Is anything growing? Is it getting darker? Does anything itch or bleed? Do you have a sore that won't go away? If any of these things are happening, then you need to bring it to the doctor's attention.

SCOTT: Some great advice. And I don't want to forget to mention that Jessica has created an incredible line of skin-care products. So, check 'em out on her website, www.DrJessicaWu.com.

DR. WU: Thanks, Scott.

BEAUTY IS more about being a good person and the way you carry yourself rather than your outside looks.

SCOTT: Let's end with everyone's thoughts on becoming your most beautiful self.

DR. WU: I think it all starts with beautiful skin because your skin is what you present to the world. Your skin, your face, your hair—it's all on display. Also important is confidence. Whenever you make me up, Scott, you make me feel so confident. You can't inject that, you can't take a pill for that, but having confidence is beautiful.

MARLEY: Beauty is more about being a good person and the way you carry yourself rather than your outside looks.

MAUREEN: I would agree completely with my beautiful daughter. So now you're all fully aware that taking care of your skin is serious stuff. You can't expect to have great skin unless you make wise, skin-sensitive choices. All of the beautiful women in this book are a testament to that. Be sure to check out their skin-care regimens, including their approach to diet and exercise. And while we haven't yet figured out how to reverse the aging process, we have identified plenty of things within our control that can not only slow down the aging process, but also enhance the health of our skin overall.

The best part is, in addition to looking healthier and learning about better makeup application, having great skin is also an amazing confidence booster. And that's perhaps the most important ingredient for becoming the best possible version of your sassy self!

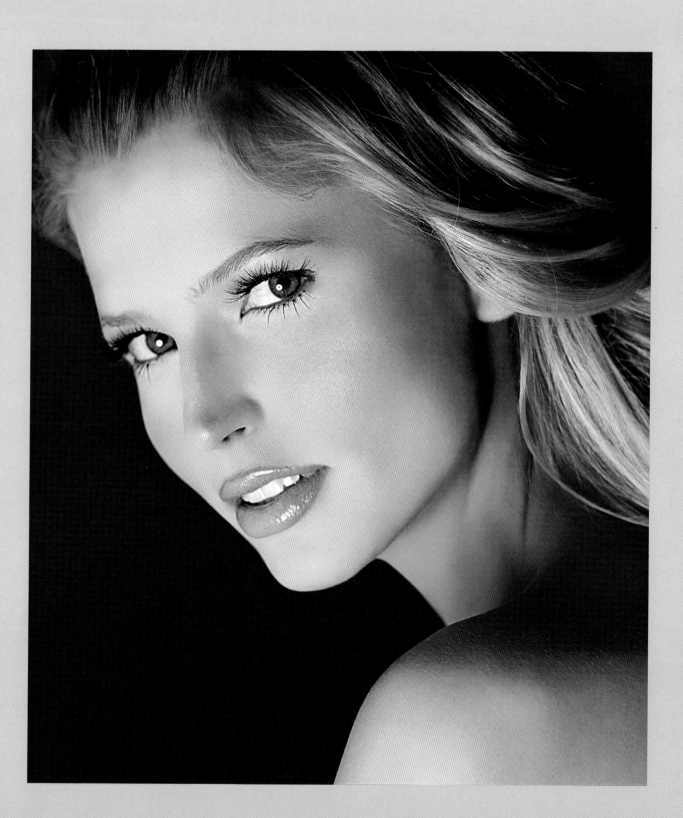

Transformations

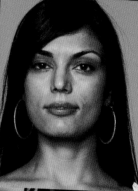

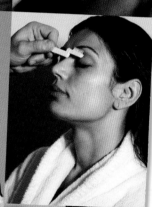

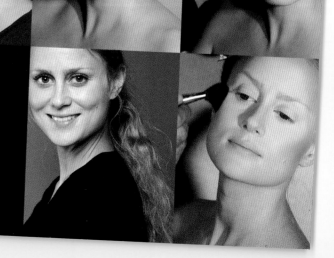

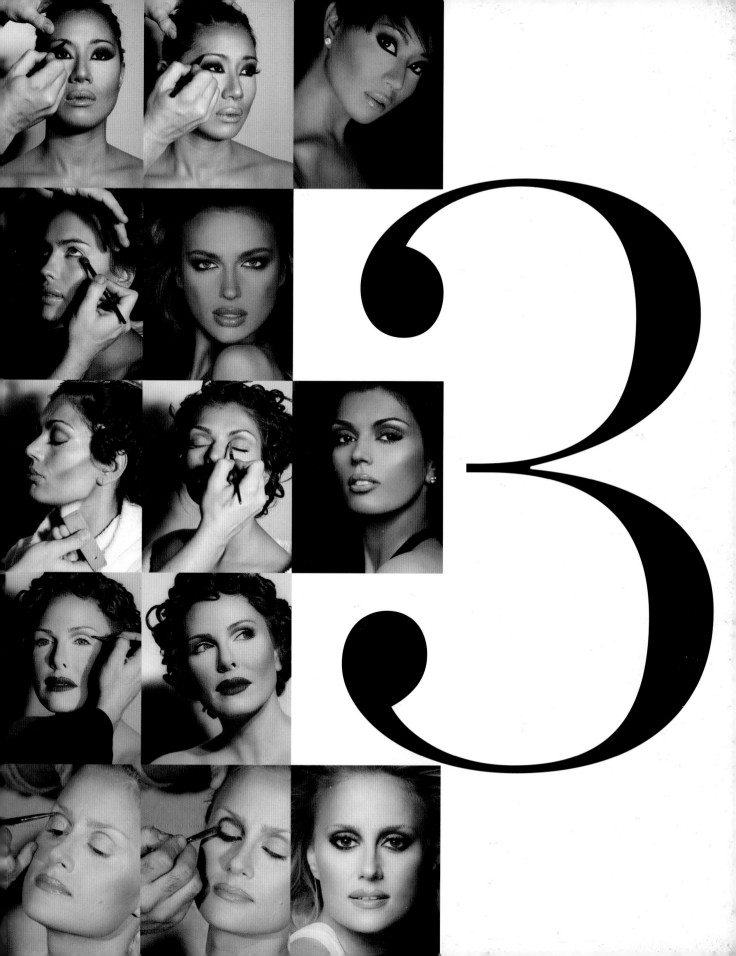

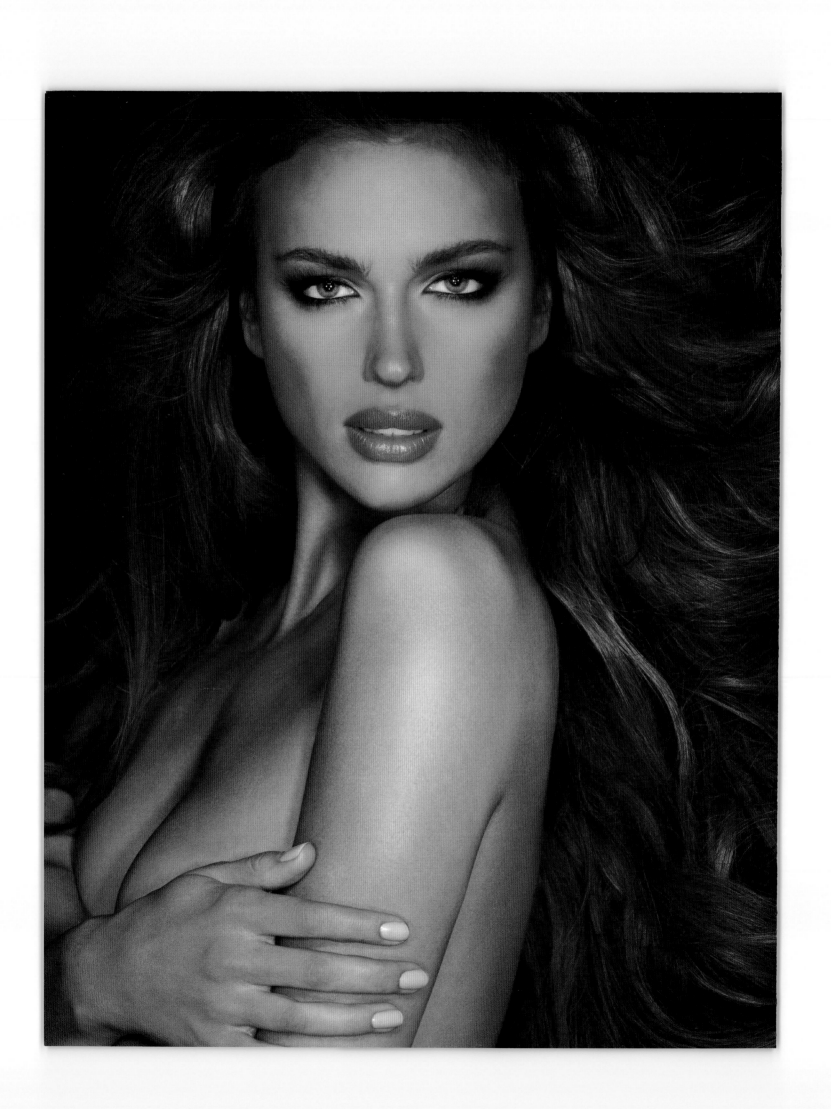

Irina:
Using Bronzer and Highlights to Create a Sun-Kissed Glow

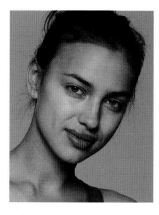

There's no denying the fact that Irina is a sexy woman. You feel her sensuality the moment she walks in the room. And that's why she's the current Guess jeans model—because she knows how to sell adventurous sex. Irina has entered the ranks of supermodels Claudia Schiffer, Anna Nicole Smith, and Eva Herzigova. But what people don't see when looking at her print image is that in addition to her apparent beauty and sex appeal Irina also has an incredibly goofy side. She and I have worked together on several different ad campaigns, and whenever we get together, much laughter is involved. She's a woman who is comfortable in her own skin—whether her clothes are on or off—and she's a great example of someone who is aware of who she is and what her power is. And that's what this book is about: the power of owning your beauty.

Scott + Irina Talk ...

SCOTT: When modeling for products like Guess jeans and lingerie, you usually have to show a lot of skin. Are you ever uncomfortable in front of the camera being so bare?

IRINA: Actually, I know that for some models, showing skin is a bit hard, but I love to work out, so I feel good about my body. Especially when I have sexy makeup and big hair: It gives me something for the shoot and helps bring something to the picture. And people are usually looking more at the face and hair than at your clothing (or lack of). So no, I don't ever feel shy or uncomfortable in front of the camera.

SCOTT: How do you stay in such good shape?

IRINA: I work out with my trainer about three to four times a week. He has a special program for me where I don't use weights. I use the weight of my body or I use very light weights, like books. I don't have any particular diet. I love to eat. I eat cake and this kind of high calorie food all the time. I think it's all about

(continued on page 163)

Creating Irina's Look

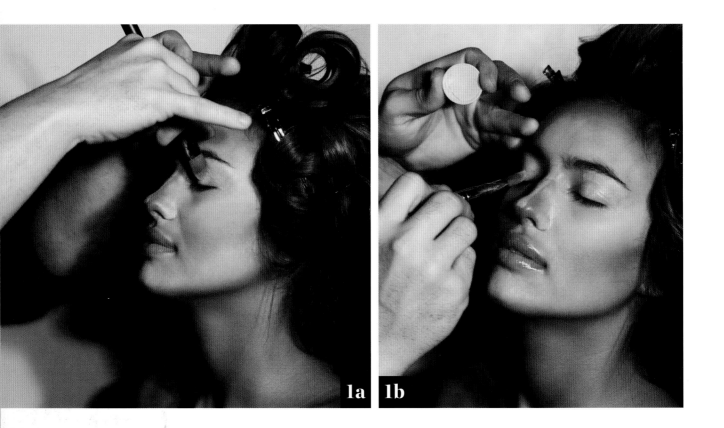

1a 1b

Tip You can put some contouring underneath the tip of the nose, to give the illusion of shortening the nose.

In my mind, Irina is a cross between a James Bond girl and Japanese anime. There's something fantastical about her. I didn't want to change Irina's look as much as I wanted to create a look worthy of an Olivia de Berardinis pin-up!

(continued from page 161)

1 Contouring, concealer, and foundation

Even though I was going for a warm, tanned look for Irina, I still needed to make sure her face had dimension and light. Looking tan isn't achieved simply by putting on a darker shade of foundation on the face. Using only one color has the effect of flattening out the face and making it look too dark. A facial tan still requires adding brightness and depth underneath the foundation first. **(a)** Using light strokes and a goat hair brush, I applied contouring (dark) cream: • Underneath the jaw line • Underneath the cheekbones • Down the sides of the nose • Underneath the tip of the nose • At the inner eye where the bridge of the nose meets the brow bone • At the top of the forehead **(b)** With shorter brushstrokes, I used a concealer brush and applied highlighting (light) concealer: • Under the eyes • Down the tip of the nose • In the middle of the forehead • At the center of the chin • On the brow bone • Covering the eye (except at the inner eye where I wanted to keep some depth) **(c)** I wanted to give Irina a warm, tanned appearance, so I applied Body Bling all over her body. You can see how much lighter the face is than the body, so the foundation is about marrying the face and body together. **(d)** I used a separate goat hair brush and applyied a light caramel-colored foundation on her face that was one shade lighter than the color of her body but one shade darker than her natural skin tone. I moved the brush in small circles to delicately blend on top of the contouring and highlighting. *Remember: Anytime you're building your face to match your body, you want to do it in layers so that your face doesn't come out looking too dark. Remember to keep more light in the center of your face and use the bronzing foundation more around the outside.*

how you eat, of course, but it's also about balancing. If you love to eat, you have to work out so your body will still look great.

SCOTT: What do you think is your best trait?
IRINA: I think that if I really, really, really want something, I can get it. It doesn't matter what it is, I'm going to find a way to get it. I can push myself. For me, it's never about wanting something and just dreaming about it; it's about taking the steps to get there. Many people, if something goes wrong, they'll give up. If I don't succeed, I can look at it a different way and find another way to approach it.

SCOTT: And your worst trait?
IRINA: Sometimes I can be very, very lazy. Let's say it's raining. I can talk myself out of going somewhere. But then, ten minutes later, I say, "No, I have to go." Also, I can be very moody. Just sometimes, but it's something I would like to get better about.

SCOTT: What are your interests outside of modeling?
IRINA: Before modeling, I went to music school for seven years, and I sang in

(continued on page 165)

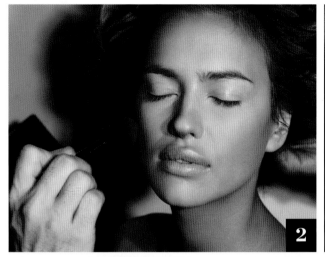

2

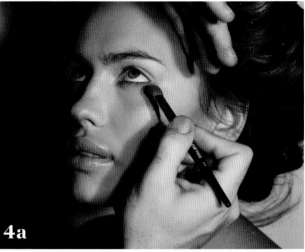

4a

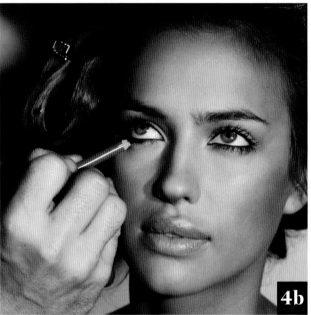

4b

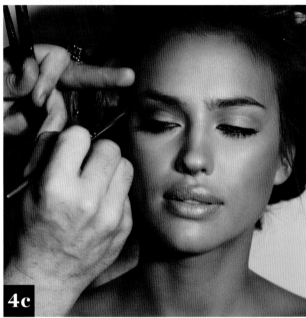

4c

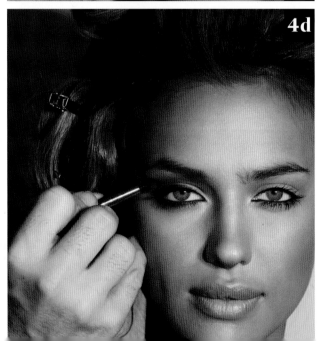

4d

Tip: Always approach blush in a very soft way, layering little by little. You can always add more, but it's very hard to remove without washing your face.

2 Cheeks

I wanted to give Irina's cheeks some color without being too overpowering. To get just the right shade, I blended two blushes together as follows. **(a)** I applied a punchy, vibrant pink cream blush to the apples of her cheeks, moving the blush brush in a circular motion. **(b)** Using a different blush brush, I layered a very vibrant peach cream blush on top of the pink, also blending in circles for a smooth, seamless finish. **(c)** To help give her cheeks more definition, I applied a very light dusting of 24-Carat Bronze highlighter on the tops of her cheekbones as well as on the apples of her cheeks for a fine sheen.

4 Eyes

To accentuate Irina's gray-green eyes, I created a smokier look by surrounding her eyes with deep rich color. **(a)** I lined the inner rim of her upper and lower lids with a black Maybelline eye pencil. **(b)** I curled her lashes and used tons of black mascara. **(c)** I surrounded her eyes with a rich chocolate-brown eye shadow. I applied it into the crease, above the crease, and underneath the eye. **(d)** With a different eye shadow brush, I went over the top of the brown eye shadow with a black eye shadow to create a smoky effect. The black by itself would've been too harsh, so I muted it by first applying the chocolate brown. **(e)** Finally, I added lots of individual false eyelashes on her upper lid.

Tip The trick with smoky eyes, like blush, is to start slow and layer up. You can always add more if necessary

3 Setting the look

With a large powder brush, I applied a warm beige loose powder all over the face to set the look as well as to add a warm glow.

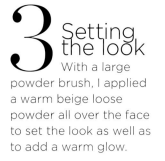

(continued from page 163)

a choir. I was one of the soloists for two years. I was a bass because I have this kind of voice [she speaks very low]. My mom is a pianist, so when I was I kid, we had a piano, and I always played with my sister.

SCOTT: Do you still sing?
IRINA: Just when I take a shower. I miss it. But it's a very hard career. With singing, you have to really be into it and you don't have much time for anything else. You can't drink cold drinks, you can't drink hot drinks, and you can't eat spicy food because all these things change your voice. And I'm enjoying the modeling now.

SCOTT: You're a hot model these days, working all the time. What do you think it takes to stay competitive in the industry?
IRINA: I think you have to always be yourself. There are always so many people around and other models, so you have to be really natural. And of course, you have to be very strong and not let the pressure get to you. I can't say that I'm better than another model. I just try to be myself and I really like what I do. It also helps to stay positive, which is easier when you enjoy what you're doing.

(continued on page 167)

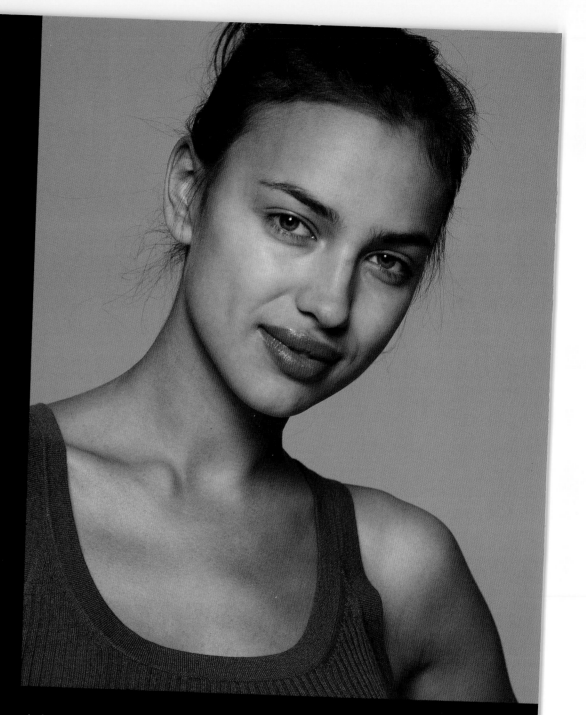

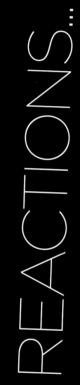

REACTIONS...

Irina's Reaction to Her Transformation

"Scott really works like an artist—the way he's using his brushes and his product. I think when he sees the person with whom he's going to work, he gets an image in his head and he creates the look he sees on you, like he is creating a painting. I wouldn't say he changed my face, even though he could if he wanted to. Scott wants you to look the same, only more gorgeous. He wants it to look natural, so he made me beautiful by enhancing what I already have."

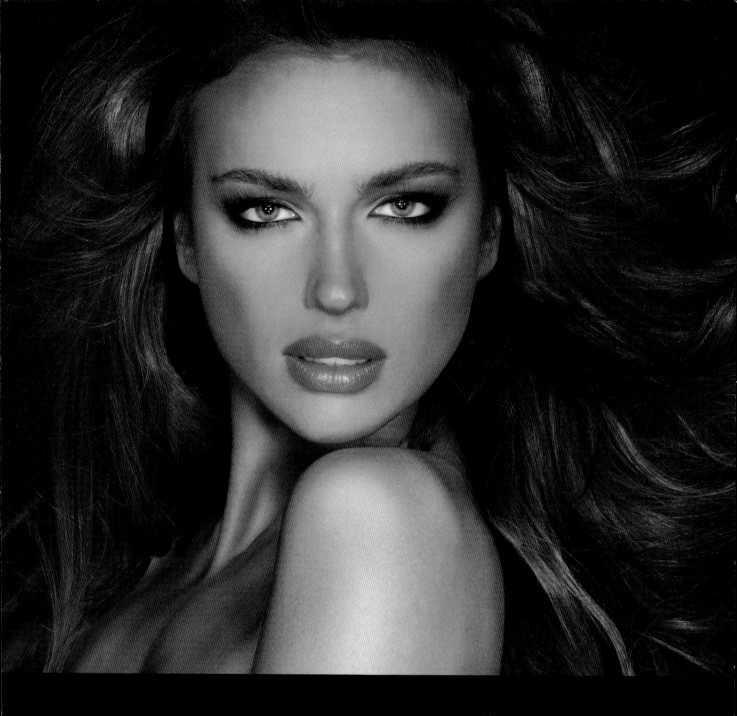

"Scott also has great energy. When it comes to makeup artists, you
want the people who touch your skin to have a great energy and
to be fun and easygoing. Scott is one of these kinds of people,
which is very rare. Also, what I love about his makeup is when he's
finished, you look healthy. Some makeup can make you look old.
But his product is very light, which is good for the skin. With Scott,
he really made my face glow, but he also made me feel very sexy
just by the way he made me feel so beautiful."

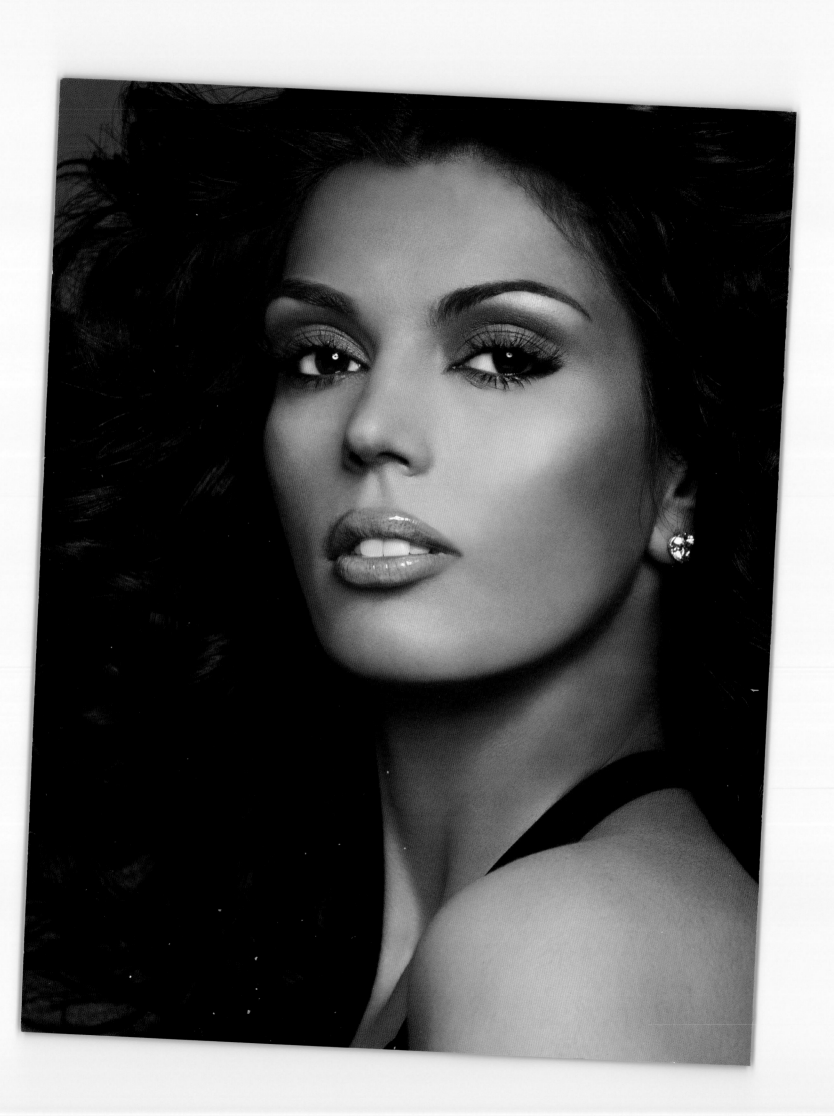

Sonia:
Going Soft and Sexy with Shimmer Highlights

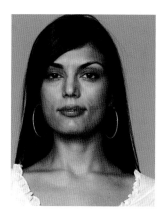

Sonia possesses a remarkable inner strength which compliments her strong, dark features. Originally from New Delhi, India, Sonia has a quiet confidence that allows her to talk easily and without conceit about herself and her approach to beauty. She starts each day with her yoga practice and peppers her conversation with phrases like "Something I deeply follow" and "I strongly believe." She seems at peace with herself and her place in the world.

Sonia also thinks like an entrepreneur. When I asked her about her skin-care regimen, Sonia told me she uses a special mask that was her own secret recipe. She wouldn't tell anyone what was in it because she plans to eventually mass market it herself. And I believe she will. Inspired by the book *The Alchemist*, by Brazilian author Paulo Coelho, Sonia states matter-of-factly that "if you want something, and you work towards it, the whole universe comes together to bring it to you."

Sonia's eyebrows are a dominant facial feature. I knew I had to start there because she had crazy brows: One was straight and the other was arched.

SCOTT: Who's plucking your eyebrows?
SONIA: Some random Indian chick off Newark Avenue [meaning herself].

SCOTT: Well, she has to be stopped. They're two different shapes.
SONIA: I know.

SCOTT: You have a very dark, thick brow, so we need to talk about how to maintain them, without plucking. I recommend using an eyebrow razor.
SONIA: Where do you get one of those?

SCOTT: You can get them at any pharmacy. It's also good for any other kinds of facial hair. So, I'm first going to clean up those brows because I want the focus to be on your eyes.
SONIA: I like my eyes, except in the morning when they are puffy. And I like my cheekbones.

(continued on page 173)

Creating Sonia's Look

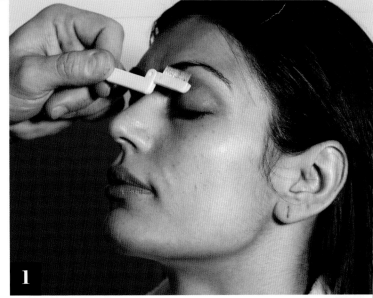

1

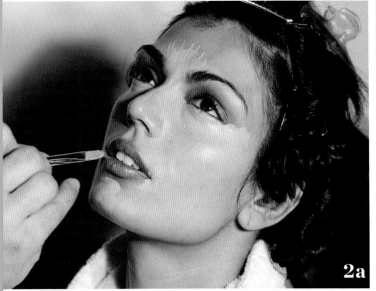

2a

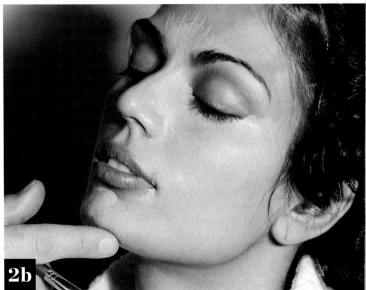

2b

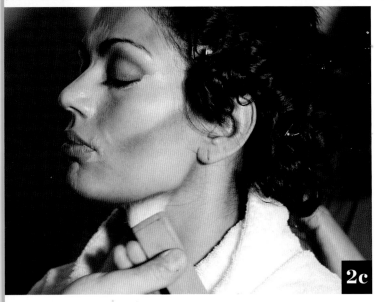

2c

Tip Yellow concealer cancels out the darkness in darker skin tones better than white or beige-colored concealer, which tends to turn gray-blue on darker skin.

Sonia's beautiful dark features and strong jaw line give her a harder look.
I wanted to soften her up for a more sensual, feminine appearance.

(continued from page 171)

SCOTT: Your eyes and cheekbones are your strongest area. You also have a pretty mouth, but that shouldn't be the main focus.
SONIA: I have a very square jaw line.

SCOTT: Yes, it's strong and gives you an angular look, so we're going to do things to soften it. Soft is more sensual, sexier. And you have the body to pull it off. What do you do for diet and exercise?
SONIA: Exercise is something I'm strict about because I believe it is very important to have discipline in your life. I work out four times a week. And I love doing sit-ups. I often compete with some cops who live in my building to see who can do more sit-ups. Other than that, I walk outside. I prefer to be out in nature. Weekday mornings, I also do yoga. It helps to release any negativity, so I start my day with clean, positive energy.

(continued on page 175)

1 Eyebrows

Sonia's eyebrows—which were slightly crooked—were a dominant feature on her face. So that's where I started for creating her softer look. **(a)** I trimmed Sonia's eyebrows with scissors and a razor comb so that the hairs would lay flatter on her face. This allowed me to see the shape of the brow. **(b)** I then began tweaking—two hairs here, one hair there—with tweezers. **(c)** Finally, I filled in a few places with a dark brown eyebrow pencil to balance out the shape.

2 Contouring and foundation

I used a yellow okra (think mustard) concealer on Sonia, since her skin tone is warm. I typically use yellow concealer on women with dark or Mediterranean skin tones: Indian, Brazilian, African American, Hispanic, Italian, or Greek. I also applied contouring foundation to help round out her face, creating a more oval-shaped face. **(a)** Using a concealer brush, I applied yellow okra highlighting concealer: ● Underneath the eyes ● At the sides of the nostrils ● From the forehead down the bridge of the nose ● On the center of the chin ● On the sides of the mouth **(b)** Using a goat hair brush, I applied a contouring (dark) foundation: ● Underneath the cheekbones ● At the jaw line ● At the inner eye where the bridge of the nose meets the brow bone ● At the temples ● At the top of the forehead where the hairline meets the skin **(c)** Using a separate goat hair brush, I applied a very warm yellow foundation on top of the contouring and highlighting. I moved the brush in a soft, circular motion for optimal blending.

Tip Eyebrows are a prominent feature on the face so give them some love. I recommend using a razor instead of plucking with tweezers to make them lay flat. Eyebrows that lie flat appear smoother than those that don't. When using a razor comb, lift the eyebrow with the razor and turn in the opposite direction. Always put a comb underneath the razor to avoid taking away too much hair.

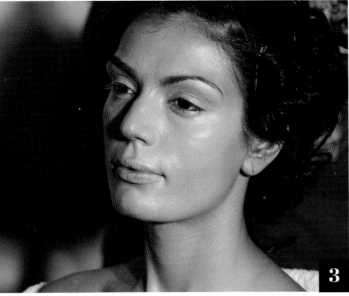

3

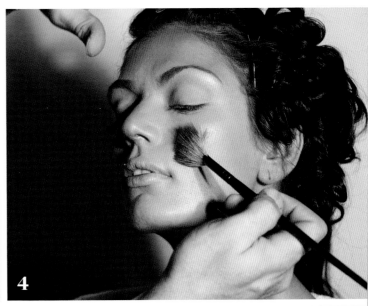

4

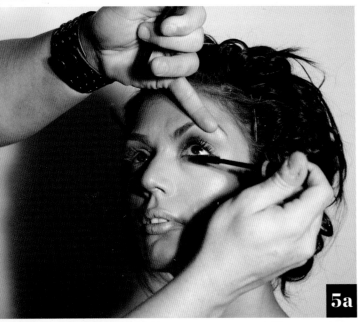

5a

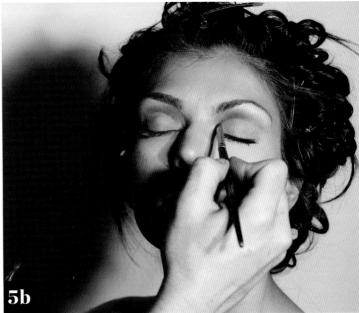

5b

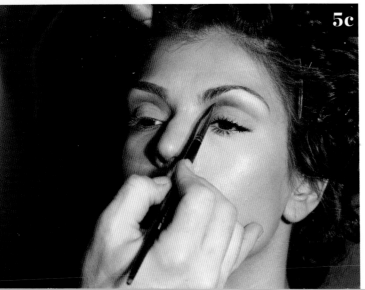

5c

Tip Shimmer highlight creates light and bone structure. You can "move" the cheekbone based on where you put your shimmer highlighter because shifting where the light reflects on the face gives the illusion of moving bones.

3 Cheeks

Using a brush blush, I applied a peachy-pink cream blush on the apples of Sonia's cheeks. I moved the brush in small, circular strokes and thoroughly blended for a seamless look.

4 Highlighting

When highlighting Sonia's cheekbones I applied the Shimmer Highlight slightly higher than her natural cheekbone to draw the eye to a different point on her face. This trick gives the illusion of softening Sonia's square jaw.

5 Eyes

Sonia has wide-set eyes, which extend even further at the outer corner, so I wanted to balance the eyes with the rest of her features. **(a)** I put smoky-gray eye shadow in the crease of her eye and slightly above. I applied it darker at the center of her eyelid, which was even with the outside corner of her mouth. **(b)** I added a light dusting of Empirical Gold eye shadow over the whole lid for a bit of subtle glamour without it looking too "Vegas showgirl." **(c)** Continuing to balance with black mascara, I applied the heaviest portion in the middle of her upper and lower lashes and less on the outside and inside corners of her eyes. **(d)** Instead of rimming the whole eye, I added a small bit of soft brown eyeliner only to the inner corners of her eyes. This helped give the eye some definition without looking overbearing or creating a heavy under-eye. **(e)** I completed the eyes with some false eyelashes. I decided to use individual lashes simply to fill in and compliment her real lashes. I avoided putting dark eyeliner around her eye, which is a more stereotypical look on an Indian woman. Remember, you want the focus to be on the eyes, not on the eye makeup.

6 Lips

Working with Sonia's normal coloring helped create full, natural-looking lips. **(a)** I applied a peachy-pink color on Sonia's lips that matched the inside color of her lips. **(b)** I finished off with a translucent shimmery pink gloss.

7 Setting the look

Using a powder brush, I set the makeup with a light dusting of translucent powder so as not to change the color of the foundation and the blush.

(continued from page 173)

SCOTT: How about diet?
SONIA: I eat whatever I want but in moderation. I stay away from all fried food.

SCOTT: How do you stay so disciplined?
SONIA: I just believe a lot. When you have faith, you can put your focus on trusting instead of worrying, and this allows you to be good to others. That's how I think a person becomes beautiful day by day. I also think it's about making conscious decisions. You have to believe that you are the most important person and everything you do to your body makes a difference.

REACTIONS...

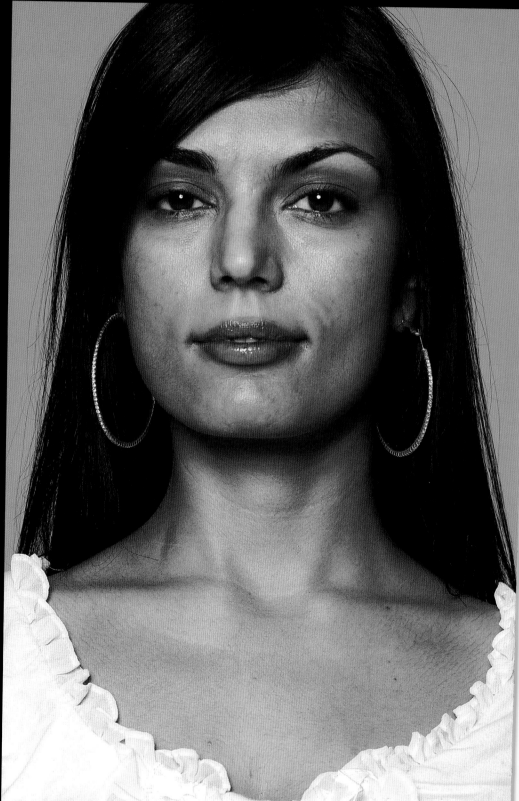

Sonia's Reaction to Her Transformation

"Scott really paid attention to my individual features and brought out the best of me, as opposed to a preconceived image of me. I never knew I should use a yellow concealer under my eyes, which blended better and enhanced my skin tone more. And the way he shaped my eyebrows... wow! My arch is so much cleaner, and they're finally even! I went right out and bought a razor comb."

"The day after I met with Scott, I experimented with some of the tricks I learned from him and when I walked into work, I got so many compliments. Overall, I think my look is much smoother and fresher. I can't say enough of what a great experience it was for me."

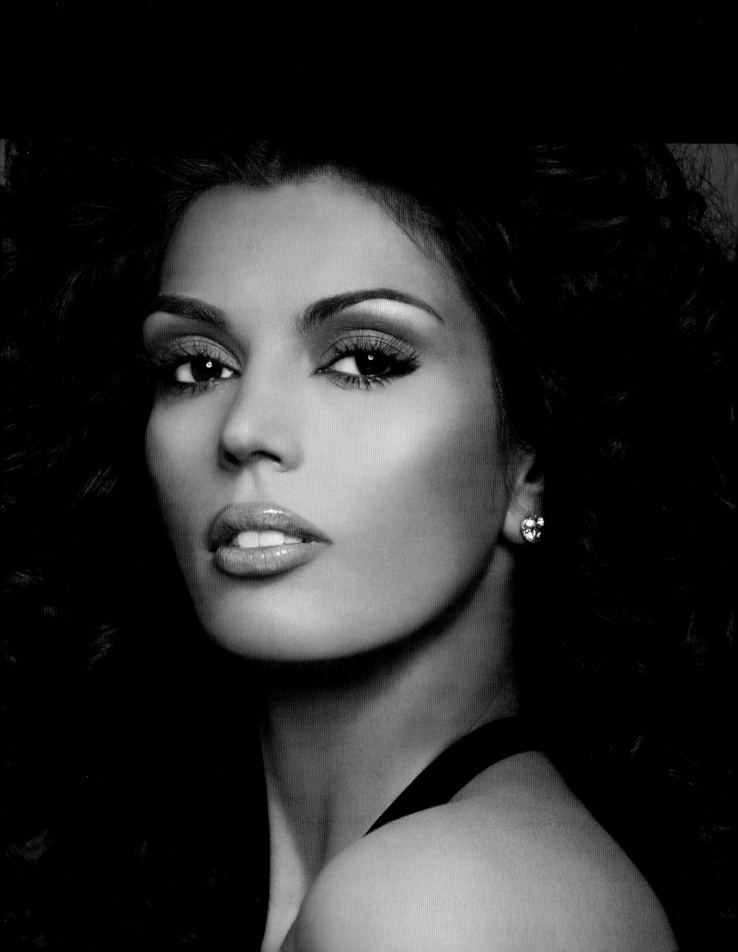

Beauty of whatever kind, in its supreme development, invariably excites the sensitive soul to tears. —Edgar Allan Poe

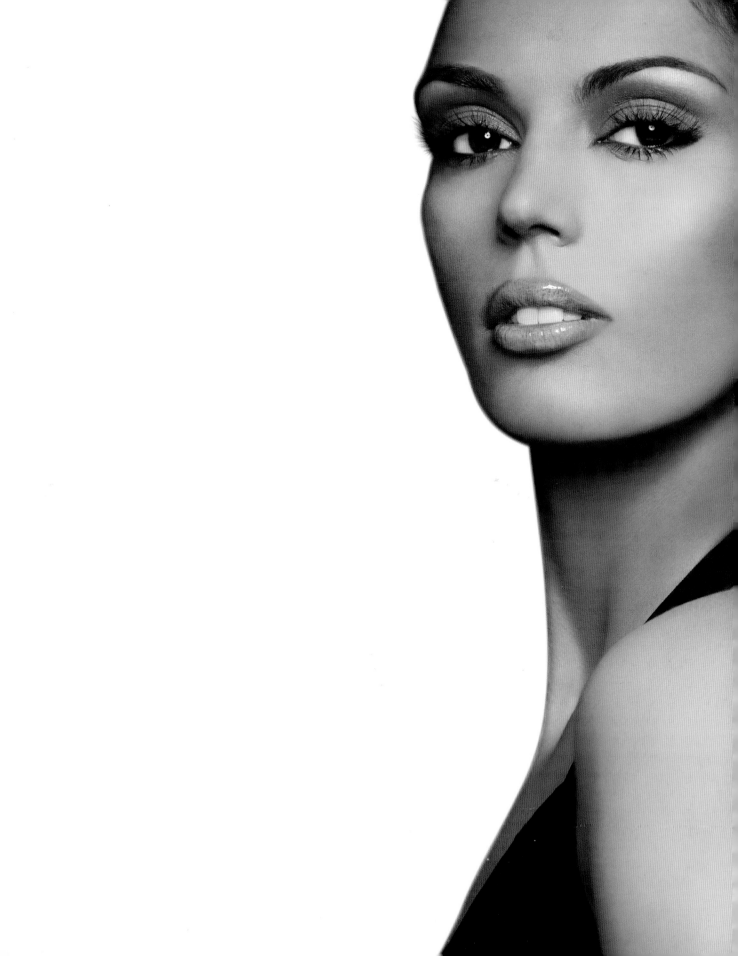

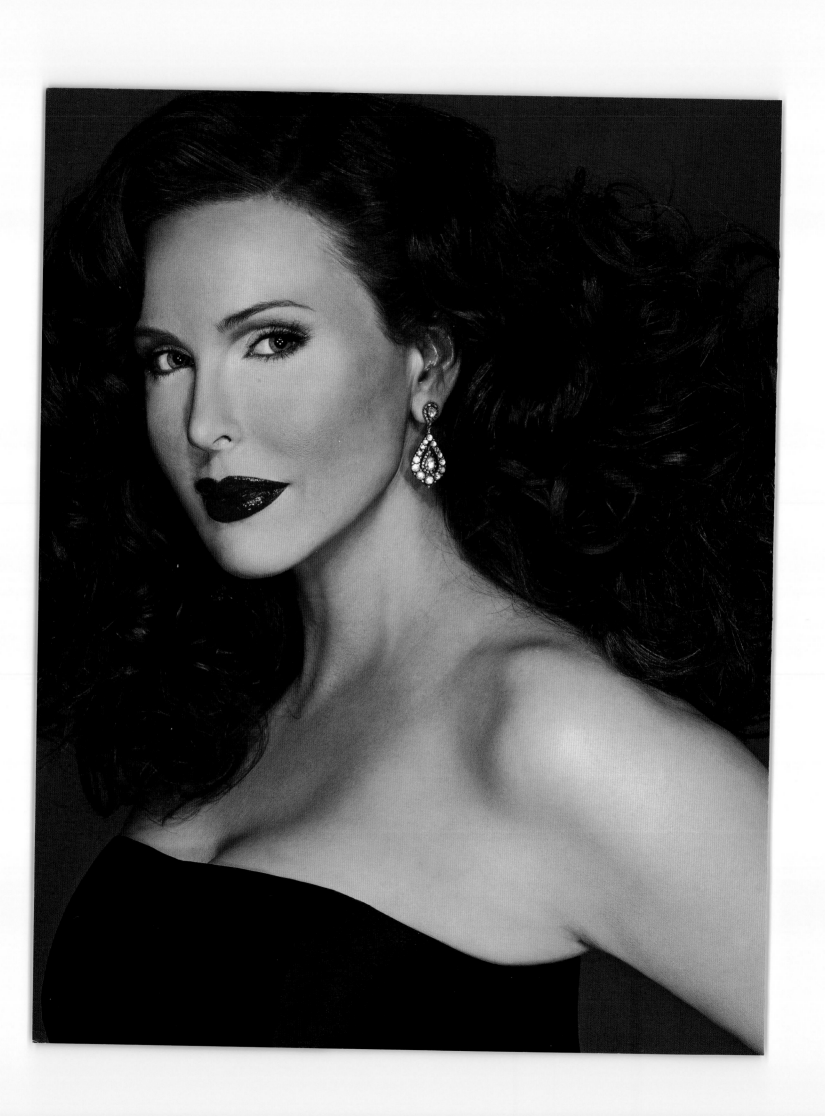

Sage:
Embracing the 1940s Glam Look

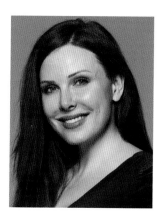

Sage knows how to turn a personal challenge into a tremendous opportunity. Having battled weight issues as a young girl, she now has a very healthy career as a plus-size model. On the board for Hearty Girls, Healthy Women, a nonprofit organization based in Maine, Sage is helping to raise awareness for the organization and advises young girls who are struggling with eating disorders and body image issues. As she puts it, "Just because you're larger doesn't mean you can't feel good about yourself and your body." It's this kind of self-respect that makes Sage all the more radiant.

In the course of our conversation, Sage told me she loved classic films of the 1930s and 1940s, Hollywood's Golden Age, which was something we had in common. She wistfully spoke of "that old Hollywood glamour" and wondered how it would feel to look like a star of that period. I decided to show her. The result was a 1940s glam look worthy of the red carpet—in any decade.

SCOTT: You began modeling when you were a teenager?

SAGE: That's right. I started modeling at fourteen, after I won a trip to Paris on the television talk show, "Good Day L.A." I ended up working as a model out of Los Angeles, and I had a lot of success in one year, but I couldn't keep my weight down. It's the classic story of a girl eating only 750 calories a day for a year, doing exactly what she was told...and it led to all sorts of health issues. So, I quit modeling, changed high schools, and eventually graduated from Sarah Lawrence College with a degree in comparative literature and theatre studies. Eventually I fell back into modeling, only this time for the plus-size division of an agency. I love plus-size modeling because it allows me to travel constantly. I'm also writing a book on body image to share my experience. I didn't know that what I was doing at fourteen was considered extreme dieting or anorexic behavior. And I really wish somebody

(continued on page 183)

Creating Sage's Look

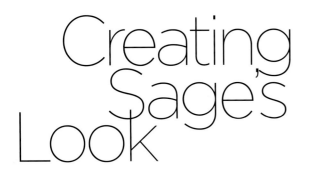

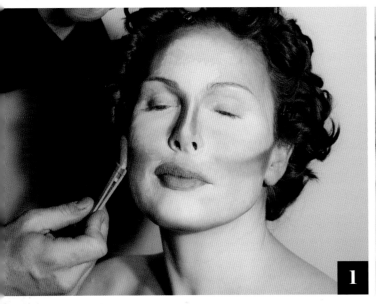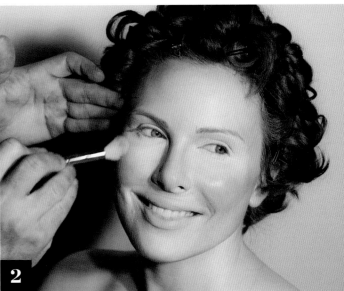

Tip When you get flush, you're blushing from underneath. So you want to mimic this natural blush when putting on your makeup.

Tip When highlighting try to put the lighter color where the sun might hit your face. Lightening these areas helps to draw the eye to these parts of your face.

I wanted to give Sage the full effect of feeling like a 1940s Hollywood starlet, so I approached her transformation the same way they might have back then—right down to the pin curls.

Keep in mind that some of the makeup you see here is exaggerated for photography purposes. I'm not suggesting you use this much when putting it on yourself. Definitely go subtler for everyday purposes.

1 Contouring, concealer, and foundation

Sage's face was on the rounder side, so I wanted to added greater contrast to create more angles and definition in her face. **(a)** I used a goat hair brush and applied contouring (dark) foundation: • Underneath the jaw line • Underneath the cheekbones • Down the sides of the nose • On the tip of the nose • On the forehead **(b)** Using a concealer brush, I applied highlighting (light) concealer: • Under the eyes • Down the tip of the nose • In the middle of the forehead • At the center of the chin **(c)** Using a separate goat hair brush, I applied a thin layer of pale beige cream foundation to counteract the redness in Sage's skin and give her a more cream-colored complexion. *Remember: Effective application of contouring, highlighting, and foundation is about one thing: blending. I use brushes for application, which I believe provides the smoothest blend, but you can also use sponges or your fingers. Whatever you use, just be sure to blend, blend, blend. Oh, and did I mention you've got to blend?*

2 Cheeks

I applied a peachy-pink cream blush on the apples of Sage's cheeks. I applied the blush with a brush and kept blending in a circular motion to create a more natural-looking peaches-and-cream complexion. *Remember: To find the apples of your cheeks...simply smile.*

(continued from page 181)

would've pulled me aside and said, "Look, you have an eating disorder." It would've saved me ten years of struggling with being really prejudiced against full-figured women. I had to work very hard to overcome my own bias against being a curvy woman. Now that I've embraced it, I feel really good in my own skin. It's ironic that the one thing I thought was holding me back is now the very thing that has made for such a wonderful life.

SCOTT: That's an important story about embracing who we are. So, how would you describe your eating habits now?
SAGE: I try to eat a balanced diet with lots of fruits and vegetables of different colors, because it really does reflect in your skin. I've always had issues with acne, so skin care's a real challenge. So, I take vitamins regularly to address it from the inside. I also use really natural skin-care products and use masks a couple of times a week.

SCOTT: What would you say you love most about yourself?
SAGE: I love my attitude. I haven't always had the same attitude, and I'm

(continued on page 185)

3 Lips

The distinguishing feature of the 1940s look is that of red hot lips. Sage already had nice full lips to pull this off, so a lot of reshaping wasn't necessary. **(a)** I lined Sage's lips with a Chinese red pencil, following her natural lip line. I then filled in her lip with the same red pencil to create a solid red lip. **(b)** I topped this off with a tinted amber glaze to give her lips a heavy shine.

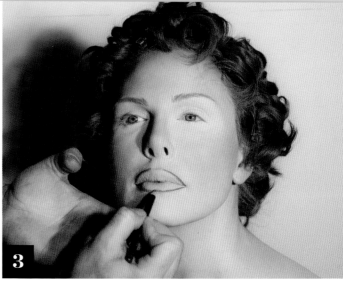

4 Eyebrows

Sage had clean, nicely shaped brows; I only needed to match them to her hair color. Matching the brow color to the hair color is an important point for redheads; otherwise, you're simply a walking billboard that says, "Hey, I colored my hair!"

For Sage, who has brown brows, I added mustard-color eye shadow to her eyebrows with an angle brow brush. This had the effect of turning her brown brows into red brows since red hair is really brown hair with a lot of gold in it.

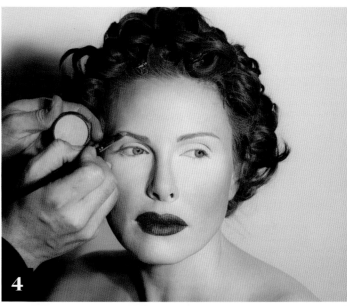

5 Eyes

Sage has fairly small eyelids, so I wanted to create a larger eyelid. **(a)** I put auburn eye shadow slightly above her normal crease. This trick helps to open up the eye and gives it a very feminine appearance. This color matched her hair color, so it would disappear into her skin and look as if she had no eye makeup on. **(b)** I blended the eye shadow into the inner corner of her eye and then faded it out toward the outside of the eye. **(c)** I also went underneath the eye with the same color, which helped bring out her baby blues.

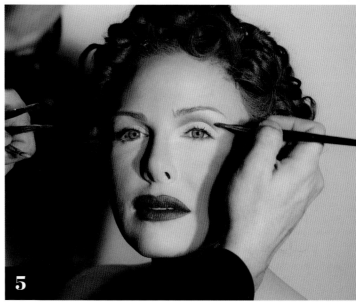

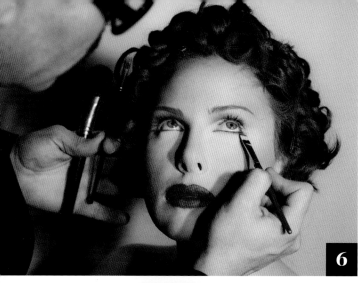

6

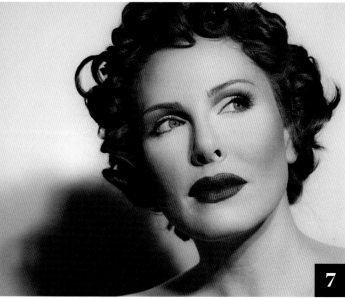

7

(continued from page 183)

6 Eye-lashes

For Sage, I used individual false eyelashes only on the outer corners to elongate her eyes. I put no lashes on the inside of her eye, to help keep the inner eye area more open. I completed the eyes with lots and lots of mascara: always.

7 Setting the look

I finished off with a nice dusting of translucent powder so as not to change the color of the foundation and the blush.

Tip Make sure you don't use a bright yellow because you don't want lemon brows!

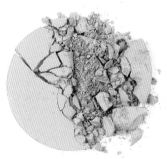

Tip If you don't have a large eyelid, you can reshape the eye with color. Simply placing your eye shadow just above the crease of your eye creates the illusion of a larger lid.

grateful for the way I have come to see things. I feel really good about my body now. I work out four times a week and either go to the gym or do yoga classes. I try to remind myself that it's a luxury to be able to have time to work out because I know a lot of people who have children or work long hours who can't really find the time for it.

SCOTT: What are your biggest beauty challenges?
SAGE: Well, of course, I don't like the acne, as I mentioned. Something else I have trouble with is redness in the skin. Especially around the nose—that's a constant concern. I'd also like to look young forever! On the other hand, I want to age gracefully, so that's another challenge I look forward to embracing.

SCOTT: You mentioned you wanted to see what it felt like to walk down the red carpet in the 1940s. Why is that?
SAGE: That was Hollywood's Golden Age, and some of my favorite films are from that era. I just always loved the way they looked. It's a different kind of glamorous than we have today.

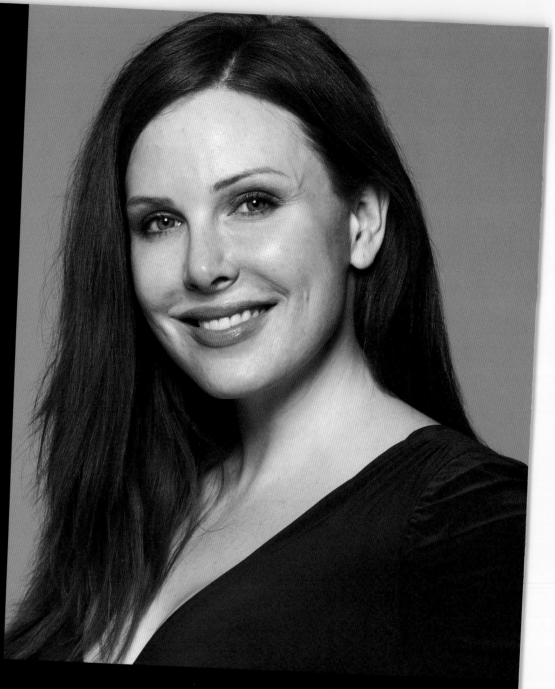

Sage's Reaction to Her Transformation

"Scott took me to a whole other place I hadn't imagined existed. I felt like a 1940s glamour puss. It's great that I now know how to do this look, and I also feel like I can integrate the different techniques into my normal routine. I mean, I love the way he did my eyes and I could do this on a daily basis."

"I'm usually so insecure with the way I do my own makeup because I have such difficulty covering blemishes and redness to the point where I practically give up. I don't usually feel the level of

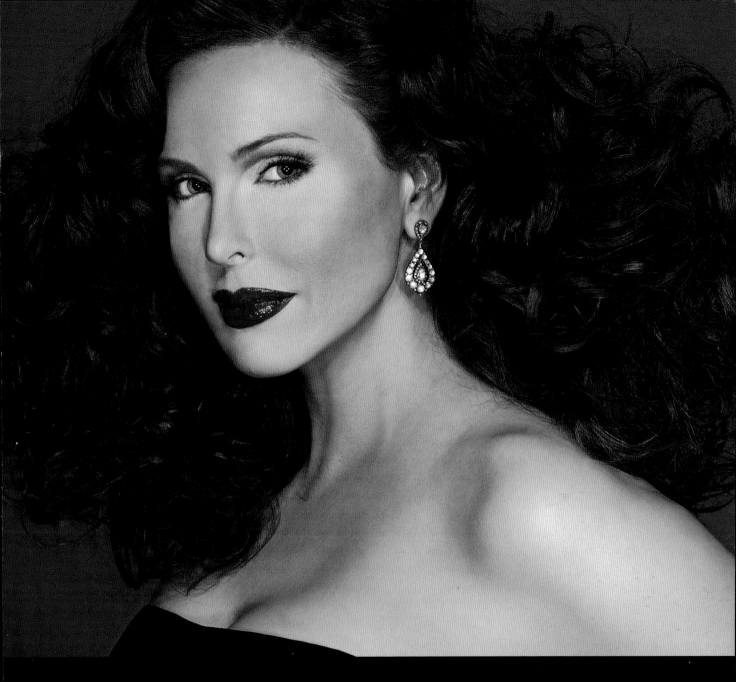

confidence that I did after Scott finished. It was a night-and-day difference. I also loved learning about what to do with my eyebrows as a redhead. I've always used a red eyebrow pencil and it made my eyebrows look brown. I've done that my whole life. But Scott showed me how to put yellow on my eyebrows instead."

"Overall the look was very showstopper, Scott definitely made me feel like a movie star!"

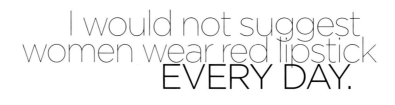

I would not suggest
women wear red lipstick
EVERY DAY.

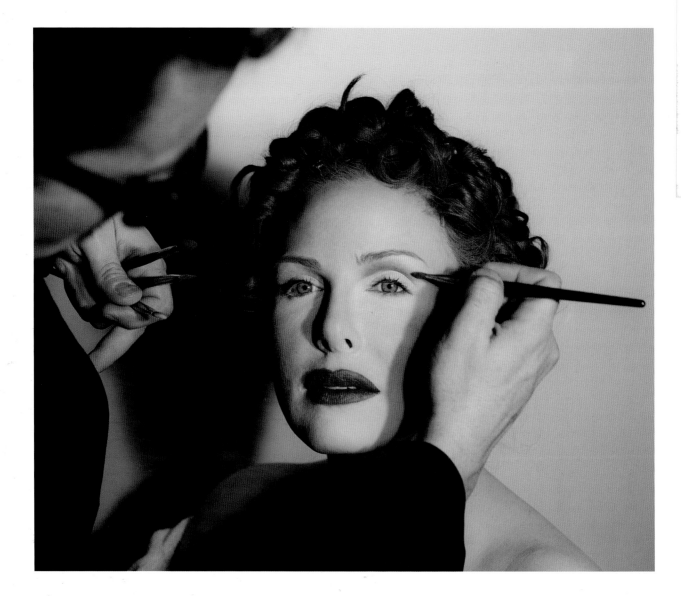

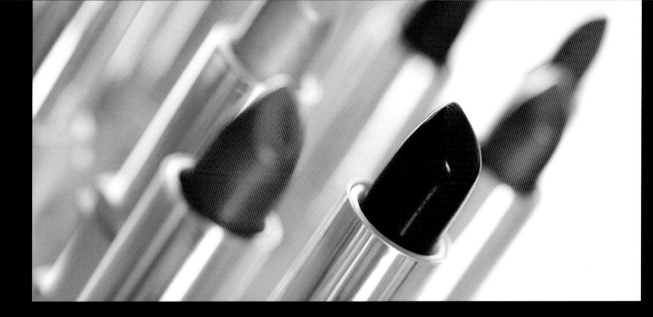

Scott Barnes on Red Lipstick: Some Dos and Don'ts

Red lipstick is used to create a very specific look. I would not suggest women wear red lipstick every day. If red lipstick is your signature thing, you'd better have a whole style and wardrobe that go along with it. Gwen Stefani is a good example. She wears red lipstick well because she has an entire wardrobe and hairstyle that support it. You can't throw on sweats with red lipstick.

DON'T wear red lipstick: • When you're wearing red—Matching red with red is tricky. It's rarely the right shade, so it usually clashes. • When you're wearing bright green. Why would you want to look like a Christmas tree? • For funerals—For some reason, women like to do the "red lipstick with a black suit" thing when they're in mourning. I feel it reads too flirty, as in, "I can't wait to bury him...who's next!" • During the day in bright sunlight— It looks too harsh.

DO wear red lipstick: • In the evening • For black-tie events • With minimal makeup on the eye (or at least the allusion of minimal makeup on the eye), like Sage • If you're a redhead.

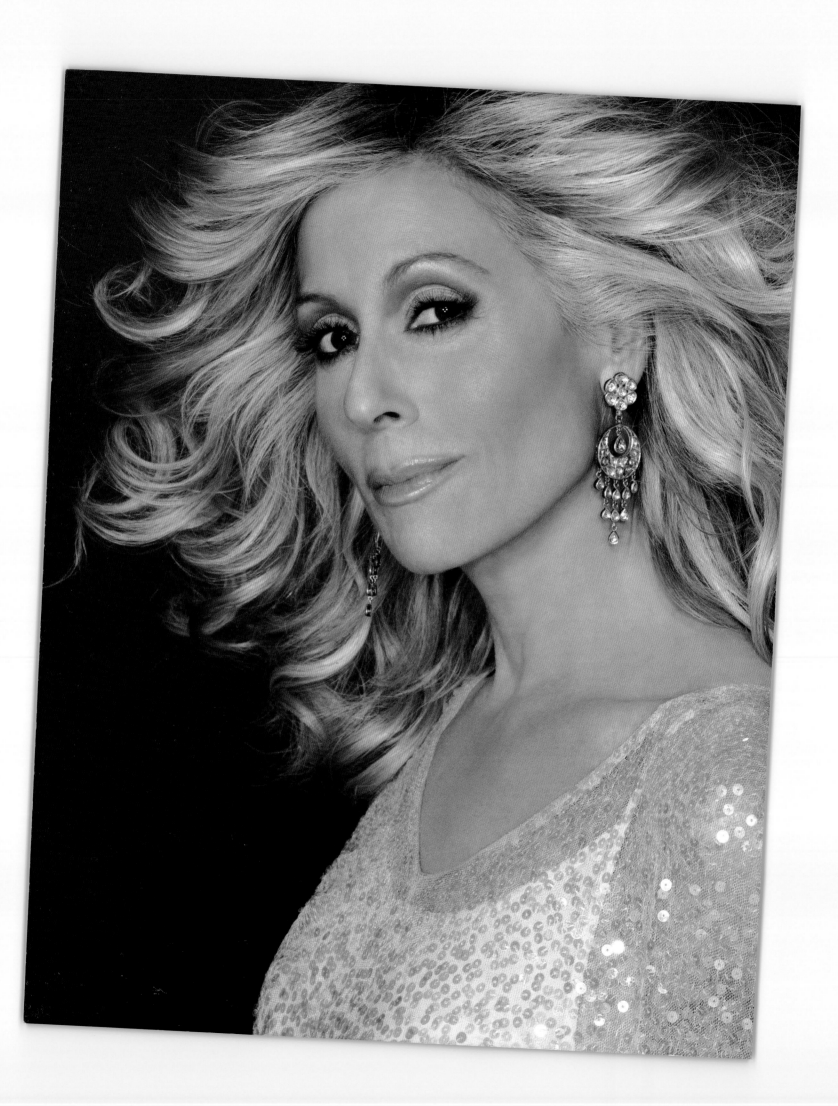

Judith Light ★

I just wanted to ENHANCE THE BEAUTY I saw when I looked at her.

Scott on Judith

Judith has an engaging magnetism, both on screen and off. While many of the characters she plays are brash, haughty types, in person she has enormous humility, gratitude, and great generosity of spirit. All these things make Judith incredibly sexy. And it's no wonder she has remained so beautiful, so remarkable, year after year.

In spite of our never having worked together before, Judith had immense trust in me as an artist. Her willingness to simply hand herself over to me revealed her own sense of confidence. It also demonstrated how well she understands the creative process. By not setting up a lot of parameters she left more room for inspiration. I didn't want to change Judith. I wasn't looking to make her into something else. I just wanted to enhance the beauty I saw when I looked at her.

Perhaps one of the things I admire most about Judith is her conviction to use her celebrity status in the service of others. She has become known as someone willing to speak out on tough issues: women's health, AIDS, and the gay and lesbian community. She spoke of her belief that "we, as human beings, all have a responsibility to be respectful of each other and our individual choices." It's this courage to take a stand that gives Judith enormous strength of character, and it resonates in every fiber of her being. It intensifies her beauty.

It's hard to define exactly why two people connect, and perhaps the why doesn't matter. The important point is that when a connection does happen, it's a rare and beautiful thing. Judith and I had an instant bond that made working together a true joy. And I knew she was somebody I wanted to have in my life for the rest of my life.

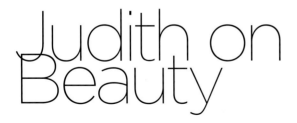

Judith on
Beauty

I try to listen from within and learn to SURRENDER.

response to that photograph. It told me that's who I long to be, a woman of substance—a woman who values experience and spirituality over the more superficial things I'm told by my society to value.

There's a kind of tenderness that we don't afford each other often enough. We need to support each other more as we go through this process called life so that we don't feel like we're struggling alone. I'm not talking about "women banding together." I'm talking about an empathetic connection as human beings. So often, we go through our busy lives encountering other individuals who make us impatient and we don't stop long enough to really take in the person whose holding up the line because, as they're digging through their change purse, their fingers don't operate as quickly as they once did or they've got something more pressing on their mind. We don't afford each other that kind of compassion,

tolerance, or generosity of spirit. I think it was Abraham Lincoln who suggested we operate as "the better angels of our nature," which goes to the question of "What is it that makes us beautiful?" It's certainly another source of beauty, doing things that make us feel beautiful. Because in the doing, we are nurturing our soul, and that's a beauty that goes beyond the physical to the real self. But if you're only listening to all the external messages, we can never become the beauty we are meant to be.

We've got to focus on the things that enlighten us, empower us, and that make us feel good about ourselves. So, I work at this. I do yoga. I walk. I eat as well as I can. I meditate. I focus on the spiritual side of my nature. I work on gratitude. I try to listen from within and learn to surrender. Fortunately, I also have a husband who thinks I am beautiful, no matter what age I am. I'm incredibly

blessed with that. And I have close friends who tell me I look terrific. It's important to listen to those people around you who really love you and who have your best interests at heart, especially when your own mind is telling you something different. And I worry less when I come across people like Scott Barnes because I know Scott will make me look as beautiful as I can feel inside. It provides a feeling of great relief, and it helps quiet those thoughts of "Oh, my neck" or "Oh, my jowls." When you look at the photograph of me, you won't see any of that. That's because Scott's an artist, a real artist, much like the old Italian masters, in the way he can make a woman look and feel beautiful.

And he makes phenomenal lip gloss.

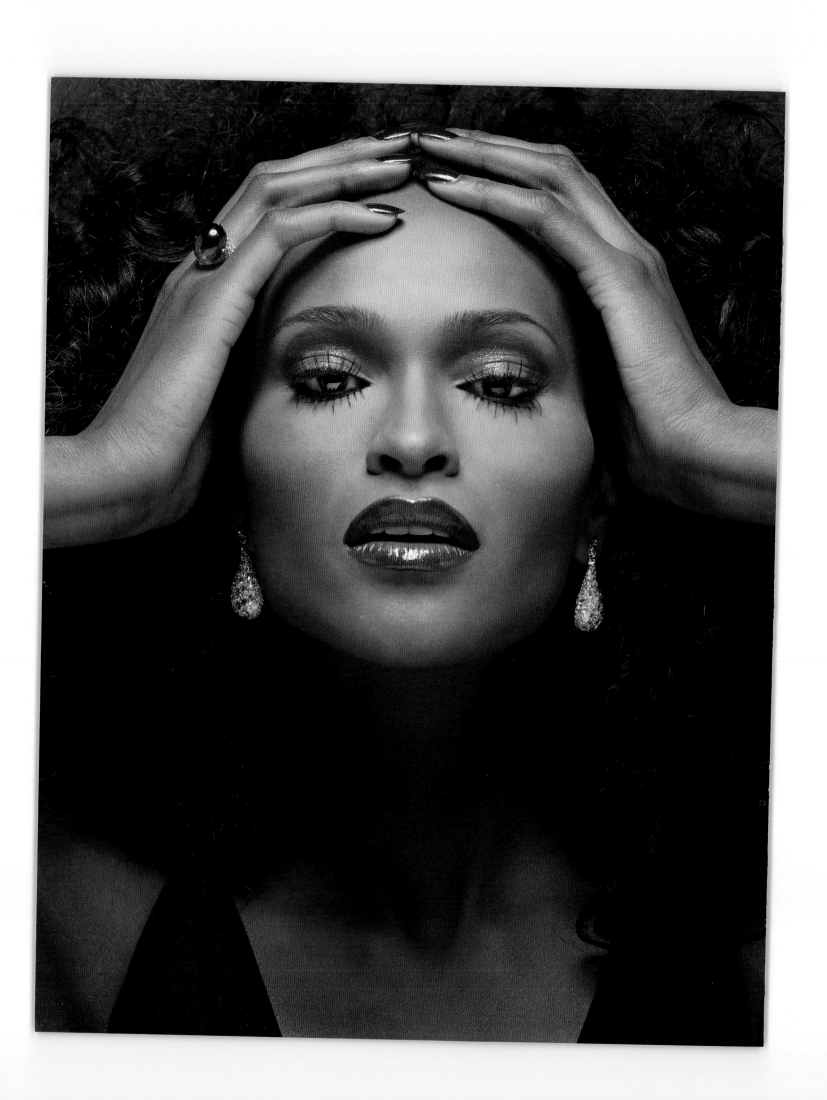

Carmelita:
Experimenting with Color for More Drama

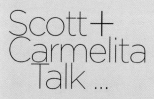

Scott + Carmelita Talk ...

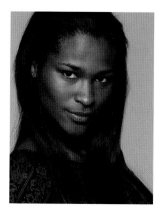

Carmelita is a Brazilian beauty. She's originally from Sao Paolo, where the rest of her family still resides. She currently models, but having recently completed a degree in biology, she's working toward becoming a veterinarian. Her love for animals is evident as her face lights up when she's talking about her boxer and two pinchers. Unfortunately, she had to leave them behind in Brazil.

Carmelita's angular face gives her a feline quality I wanted to capitalize on. I knew I needed to balance out her long jaw and reshape her hairline for a cleaner, more balanced look. Also, as beautiful as Carmelita looks naturally, I wanted to show her that she could unleash her diva within!

SCOTT: Do you ever get mistaken for being African American?

CARMELITA: Yes, and I always correct these people. Brazilian women are a mixture of races, even though they have the skin color and strong features that look similar to those of African-American women.

SCOTT: Do you have any favorite foods or drinks?

CARMELITA: A Brazilian dish: beans, rice, and meat. I like African food also and Italian. I'm not a vegetarian; I like my meat. I stay away from French fries. I eat no fried foods in general. And I drink wine, juice, tea... everything.

SCOTT: Do you like to exercise?

CARMELITA: I like to ride the bicycle at the gym, for my legs. I go to the gym, but not every day since I don't always have the time. But I walk every morning for about thirty minutes.

SCOTT: Do you like to wear makeup?

CARMELITA: Yes, but I like to wear very natural

(continued on page 197)

Creating Carmelita's Look

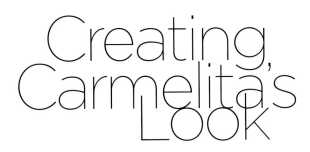

Carmelita was used to going with a natural, no-makeup look. I wanted to show her that she had room to experiment with much more color since she has so much depth to her dark skin. My goal was to create a dazzling presence that would rival any dance-floor diva.

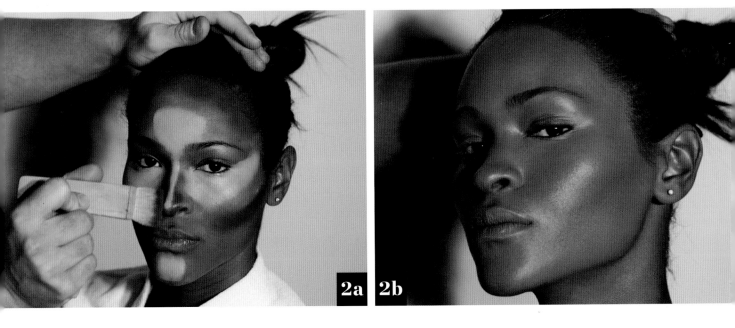

2a 2b

(continued from page 195)

1 Prepping the face

Sometimes, like in Carmelita's case, you'll want to address unwanted facial hair or an uneven hairline before beginning makeup application to achieve a cleaner, more polished look. This helps bring the focus into the center of the face, to your eyes, nose, and mouth. ● Hairline and upper lip: Using a razor comb I trimmed Carmelita's hairline to take the jagged edges off and soften the frame of her face. I also removed the fuzz from her upper lip. ● Eyebrows: Using a razor comb, I thinned and shaped Carmelita's eyebrows and then plucked a few stragglers with tweezers. *Remember: When shaping the eyebrows, always strive for minimal plucking with tweezers to avoid permanently damaging the hair follicles.*

2 Contouring, highlighting, and foundation

Carmelita's got terrific facial bones which make for great angles. So, when applying foundation, I wanted to be sure I didn't flatten out her face by using only one color of foundation. Carmelita's skin tone contains both red and yellow pigment. This combination of colors is why Carmelita has a bronzy color to her skin. Instead of trying to match one color or the other, I used both to stay as close as possible to the light and dark of her natural coloring. **(a)** Using light strokes with a goat hair brush, I applied a reddish-burgundy contouring foundation: ● At the bottom of the chin, instead of underneath the jaw line (to give the illusion of shortening the chin) ● Underneath the cheekbones ● On the sides of the nose ● At the inner eye where the bridge of the nose meets the brow bone ● At the temples ● Under the tip of the nose (This gives the illusion of shortening the nose.) ● At the top of the forehead where the hairline meets the skin **(b)** Using a concealer brush, I applied yellow highlighting concealer: ● On top of the cheekbones ● Underneath the eyes ● From the forehead down the bridge of the nose ● On the upper part of the chin (This gives the illusion of shortening the chin since the eye is drawn to where the light hits the chin.) **(c)** Using a separate goat hair brush, I applied a thin layer of bronze cream foundation on top of the contouring and highlighting. *Remember: Blend thoroughly, moving the brush in a circular motion to marry all the colors and achieve the smoothest finish. Remember: If you have dark skin, you should have two or three foundations that you can blend to create a more natural-looking foundation with greater dimension. Dark skin is never one color. When applying foundation you want to attempt to mimic the natural color of these different skin tones; otherwise, you risk flattening out your face by making it either too light or too dark.*

makeup, all organic; and not too much makeup. I like to look very natural. If I'm going out, I will put on mascara and blush and some gloss. But I find it's very difficult to buy the right blushes and shadows for my skin color, so I usually go without.

SCOTT: What do you do for skin care?
CARMELITA: For cleaning my face, I use a soft cleanser in the morning and then I put on lotion. I don't put too much on my skin because I prefer my skin to be very natural. At night, I always wash my face and put on cream too.

SCOTT: Are there things about yourself that you like or dislike?
CARMELITA: I don't like my hair, because it is so short. So, I put extensions in my hair to make it longer. You can see I have extensions in now! I think I like nearly everything else about myself. If I could change one thing, I would maybe change my butt, because it is so skinny.

(continued on page 199)

I gently pressed the powder puff over her face to SET THE MAKEUP.

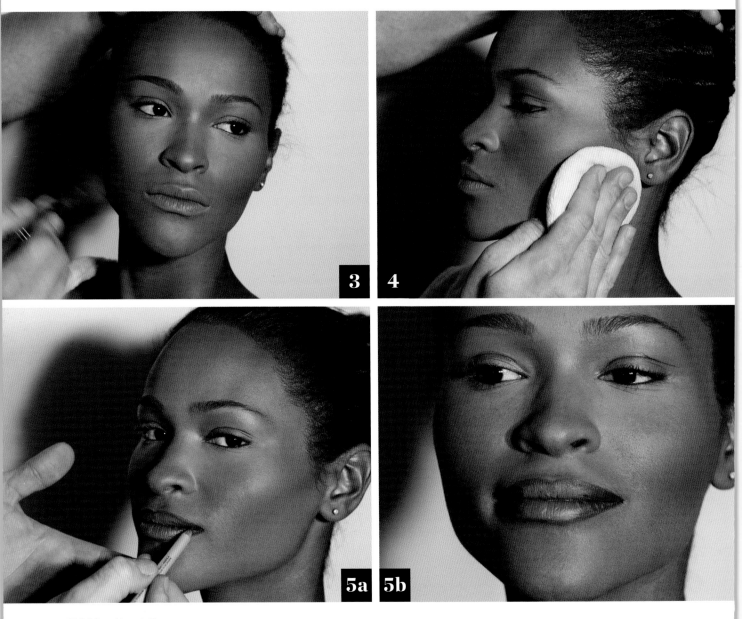

3

4

5a 5b

3 Cheeks

I applied a reddish-burgundy cream blush to the apples of Carmelita's cheeks and blended in circular strokes for a seamless transition.

4 Setting the look

As I've mentioned before, this is a very important step for creating a flawless finish. You can use either a loose powder with color or a translucent powder. I opted to use a light tan loose powder with a yellow under-tone. This helped to bring out the bronze tone in Carmelita's skin. **(a)** With a very large fluffy powder brush, I loosely dusted powder all over Carmelita's face and neck. **(b)** I tapped the excess powder from the brush onto a powder puff. I then folded the puff as though I were making a taco and smushed the powder into the puff. This trick buries the excess powder into the puff so that it doesn't end up on your face. **(c)** I gently pressed the powder puff over her face to set the makeup.

5 Lips

To select the lip liner color, I used the darkest spot of Carmelita's lip, which turned out to be close to a chocolate-burgundy color. **(a)** I lined Carmelita's lips following her lip line. **(b)** I shaded the inside inner corners of her lips to create more depth on the inside of her lips. **(c)** I later finished the lips off with lip gloss (see step 7 on page 201).

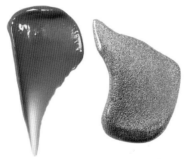

(continued from page 197)

SCOTT: Who do you consider beautiful?
CARMELITA: Beyoncé.

SCOTT: Is it difficult to be such a beautiful woman?
CARMELITA: I don't consider myself to be a pretty lady. It's only when I have makeup put on me that I think I can look pretty. Makeup can change the face so much, so if you have beautiful makeup, then you can become beautiful!

Using separate brushes
is the best way to
AVOID MIXING eye shadow
colors in their cases as well.

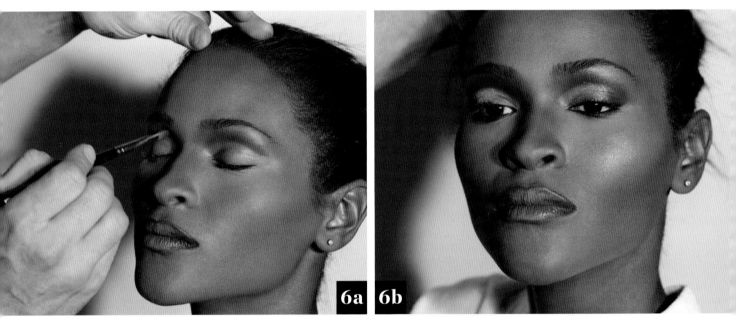

6a 6b

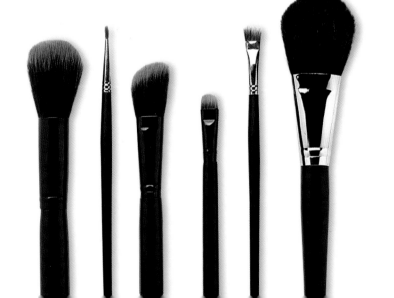

6 Eyes

I mentioned earlier that Carmelita has red and yellow undertones. I used the same reddish-burgundy that I used for contouring as an eye shadow base, creating depth and contour around her eyes. I used different eye shadow brushes for each of the following steps for cleaner application. Using separate brushes is the best way to avoid mixing eye shadow colors in their cases as well. **(a)** First I hollowed out her eye by blending the reddish-burgundy contouring powder in the crease of her eye and in the inner corner of her brow bone. **(b)** I layered a purple eye shadow right in the crease and just above it. **(c)** I added a fine line of black eye shadow using a very thin eyeliner brush in the crease for a more dramatic effect. (We're talking diva here!) **(d)** I applied the reddish-burgundy contouring shadow underneath the eye as well, using a brush with a very fine, slightly chiseled point. **(e)** I lined the eye with a black pencil to give the eye some depth, and I outlined from the middle of the lower eyelid to the middle of the top eyelid to draw the focus to her outer eye, which gave the effect of opening up her eyes. (Applying the liner towards the inside of her eyes would have the effect of "closing" her eyes slightly, making them appear smaller and closer together.) **(f)** Since we were going for high drama with Carmelita, I finished off with purple glitter on her eyelids. Just be sure not to "drip" glitter all over other areas of your face; otherwise, you'll be noticed for all that glitter on your face, not your own beauty. **(g)** I finally added some upper and lower false eyelashes for the full diva effect. *Warning: Caucasians, don't try this at home! If you apply these colors on your fair skin, it will end up looking like you were in a scary accident!*

7 Lip gloss

I finished the lips with a Black Cherry Patent Leather lip gloss.

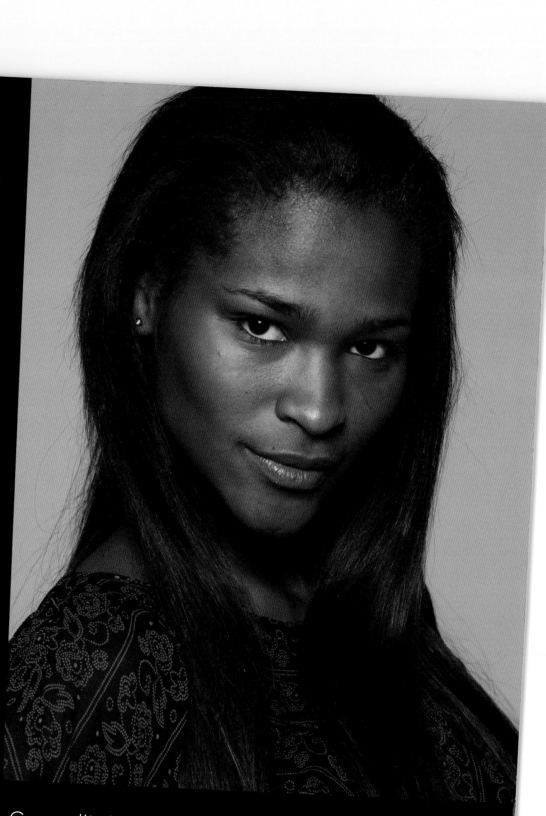

REACTIONS...

Carmelita's Reaction to Her Transformation

"I look so different! I love the makeup so much—the color of my skin, the color on my eyes, the way he made my face look not so long and skinny—everything's so, so pretty. Scott used different colors for the base of my skin. My skin color is very dark in some parts, but not in all parts. So, I've learned how to use different colors for this base instead of using just one color. This pleases me very much.

I also know now that using more color for my face, like purples or reds, is very good for me. Scott put it on my eyes, a little bit on my lips, and on my nails. Normally, I would wear black or darker colors. Now that seems boring. He also used more color in my cheeks, like red, and put black eyeliner inside my eye. It makes such a big difference to use brighter colors. This makes me feel very chic."

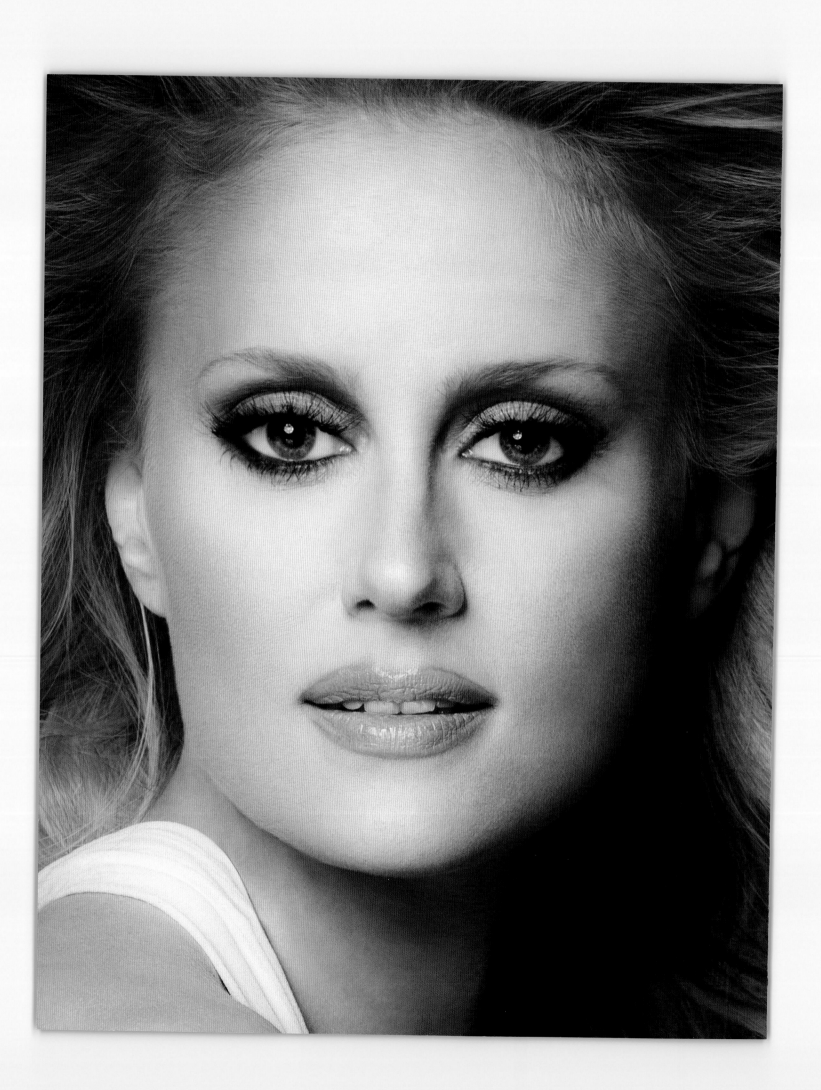

Linda:
Time-Saving Tips for the Busy Woman

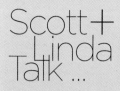

Scott + Linda Talk ...

Linda has had a big year: she got married, bought a house, and became pregnant. Weekdays, she works full time for an Italian designer in New York City. On weekends, she is fixing up the new house, and basically trying to get as much done as possible before the baby arrives. Linda doesn't slow down long enough to look in the mirror, much less devote time to a beauty regimen. Linda used to "love to play with makeup" when her life was less complicated, "but now," she told me, "I've completely let myself go."

I see too many women fall into this trap. They're juggling so many things, and they make less time for themselves. Unfortunately, they also start to feel less good about themselves, and often, their self-worth and their relationships suffer. Linda admitted she was feeling less beautiful over the past year, especially since she had gotten pregnant. My hope was that Linda's transformation would help her reconnect to her womanliness and give her a more positive self-image. As Linda transformed, it was thrilling to watch her regain a sense of her own sex appeal.

SCOTT: Is it safe to assume that given your very busy life, you have a pretty simple skin-care routine?
LINDA: Yes, it's very basic. Most mornings I wash and then moisturize. I usually buy the pharmacy brands, nothing expensive. I buy different brands, but the one brand I have been using since I was a kid is Nivea. I use their oldest facial cream, which is this really heavy, thick cream that feels almost like cold cream. It's a classic, and I use it morning, day, evening, all the time.

SCOTT: Do you ever take time out for yourself?
LINDA: Not really. I certainly don't pamper myself anymore—I rarely go get a manicure, I don't do my makeup...I feel like I've completely let myself go. I have just been overwhelmed with everything going on. I work full-time, then I got married, we bought the house, and we got pregnant...everything happened in a year. And I haven't really had time off to myself at all. It'd be nice to feel like a woman again.

(continued on page 207)

Creating Linda's Look

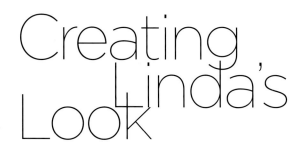

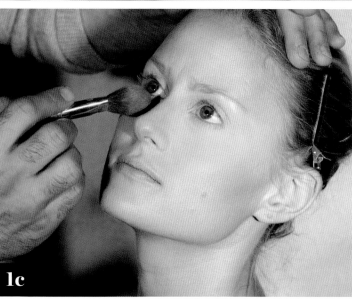

1a

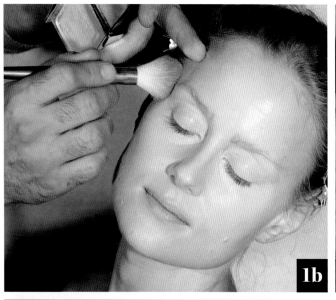

1b

1c

Time-Saving Tip

You can always spot-conceal by putting concealer only in those places where it is really needed: under the eyes, around the sides of the nostrils, and over any blemishes. Just make sure you blend these places really well. Adding a quick dusting of translucent powder on top will help with this.

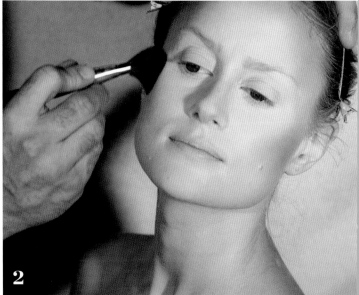

2

Just because you get married doesn't mean it's over. Just because you're having a baby doesn't mean it's over. Actually, it's just the beginning. Your priorities may shift, but you don't want to forget about taking care of yourself. Remember, half of feeling good is looking good, and looking good leads to feeling good. Putting on makeup doesn't have to be a time-consuming process. But it's worth the few minutes it takes to make yourself feel better. Here are the steps for creating Linda's look, as well as some time-saving tips.

1 Contouring, highlighting, and foundation

I did very light contouring for Linda since her coloring is so fair. **(a)** With extremely light strokes, I applied contouring (dark) foundation: • Underneath the cheekbones • On top of the forehead • At the temples **(b)** Using a concealer brush, I applied highlighting (light) concealer: • Under the eyes • Down the tip of the nose • In the middle of the forehead • At the center of the chin **(c)** Using a separate goat hair brush, I applied a thin layer of cream beige foundation, which I thoroughly blended with the contouring and highlighting for a smooth finish.

2 Cheeks

Linda's face is on the longer side, so I wanted to help shorten it some by making sure I put the blush on the apples of her cheeks. Placing the blush underneath her cheekbones would have had the effect of making her face look longer and more drawn out.

Moving the brush in a circular motion, I applied a pale-pink cream blush on the apples of her cheeks, a color that was a warmer rather than cooler pink. This color complimented her fair features with just a hint of color without being too dramatic.

(continued from page 205)

SCOTT: What do you love best about being a woman?
LINDA: I love to wear dresses. I'm a girly girl... I rarely wear jeans.

SCOTT: Where are you from originally?
LINDA: Finland. But I've been living In the United States for more than fifteen years.

SCOTT: Do you see a difference in the way women approach beauty in Finland versus here in the States?
LINDA: Yes, Finnish women don't put as much time into their appearance as American women...for better or worse. It seems like women here spend much more time taking care of themselves, focusing on things like teeth whitening.

SCOTT: What is your idea of beautiful?
LINDA: My nanny, who is now a dear friend of mine, used to say, "Many a cake is pretty on the outside..." meaning that even if the frosting looks great, it doesn't mean the cake will actually taste good. So, I learned very early that being beautiful isn't about a person's exterior. True beauty is all about how you treat other people; being beautiful is about being nice to everyone around you.

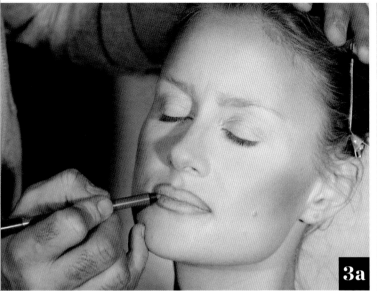

3a

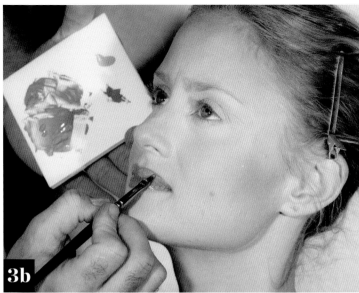

3b

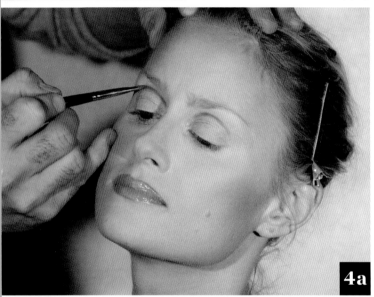

4a

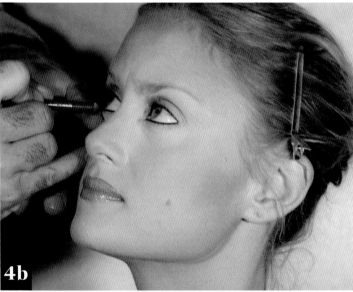

4b

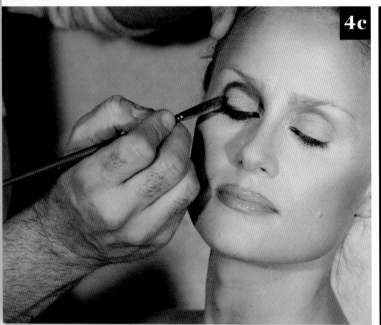

4c

Time-Saving Tip
If you've got no time to think about lip liner and color, simply go with a tinted lip gloss. A little gloss can go a long way toward giving you a fresh, healthy appearance. Never leave home without your gloss.

3 Lips

Linda has nice full lips, so it was really a matter of bringing out what she's already got and using colors that would compliment her sparkling blue eyes with a tiny bit of color. No reshaping of the lips was necessary. **(a)** I lined Linda's lips with a taupe lip liner, a color that was one shade darker than her lip color, by following her natural lip border. **(b)** I filled in with a pastel pink lipstick. **(c)** I completed with a sheer lip gloss.

4 Eyes

Linda's eyes are close-set, so I kept everything heavier on the outside corners of her eyes to give the illusion that her eyes are a little farther apart. **(a)** I covered the whole eye with cream beige foundation—the same that I used earlier on her face. This gave me a more even base on which to layer color since Linda' eyelids had touches of red pigment in them. **(b)** I applied a smoky gray eye shadow on the top lid along the outside half of the lash line. **(c)** Using this same smoky gray shadow, I filled in at the crease of the eye and on the outside half of the upper lid. **(d)** I lined the whole inside of the eye—upper and lower—with a black Maybelline pencil to really accentuate her blue eyes. **(e)** I went back in with the smoky gray eye shadow and applied a thin line of color underneath the eye. I delicately smudged the line after applying for a softer effect. I used this color to create a more sultry, smoky look for Linda. **(f)** I finished off with black mascara on both the upper and lower lashes, with an emphasis on the outside corners of her lashes to draw the eyes outward.

5 Setting the Look

Using a fan brush, I softly dusted champagne shimmer highlight on the tops of her cheekbones, forehead, and nose to add a warm overall glow to the look and followed that with a light dusting of translucent powder.

Time-Saving Tip

Eyeliner can do a lot in terms of quickly enhancing your eyes if you don't have a lot of time. The same is true with mascara. You can line the inside rim of the eye—both the upper and lower lids—and use either black or brown liner. Just be careful that you don't make it too harsh-looking, if you have time to apply only minimal makeup.

Time-Saving Tip

Simply put a tiny bit of shadow along the crease of your eye using your fingers, just to give your eyes some dimension.

Linda's Reaction to Her Transformation

"I have to say, I've never felt so glamorous in my whole life. I feel ten years younger! Also my husband looked at me in a fresh way again, and that was definitely nice. I didn't want to wash it off! So, now I've started to take a little extra time in the morning. And when I do something as simple as put mascara and liner on my eye, it makes a big difference. Just putting in that extra five minutes...and I actually had to wake up five minutes earlier just to do that one little thing...but it makes all the difference! It's true that you really do feel better about yourself if you feel like you look good. I can even feel a difference in the way that I work; I work with more confidence. I feel

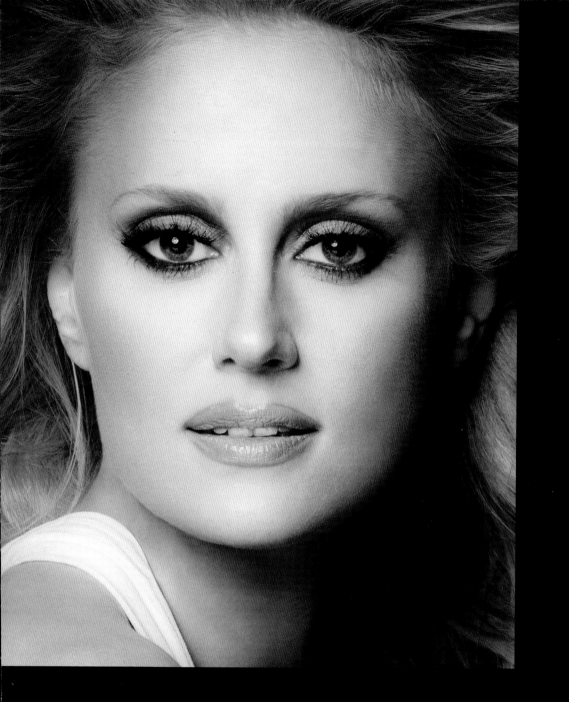

100 percent more confident with makeup on. I feel like a woman again and that's really nice. So, I think a woman should really try and make the effort. And now, if my husband and I go out somewhere, I wear a bit more makeup. A little bit goes a long way. I do it for my husband. But I also do it for myself."

"I want to say one more thing. Scott's whole 'glow' thing has always fascinated me, and it was incredible to see up close the way he applies the highlights and the lowlights. At one point he put a little bit of sheen on the tip of my nose—a shimmery highlight—and it transformed my face in a really surprising way."

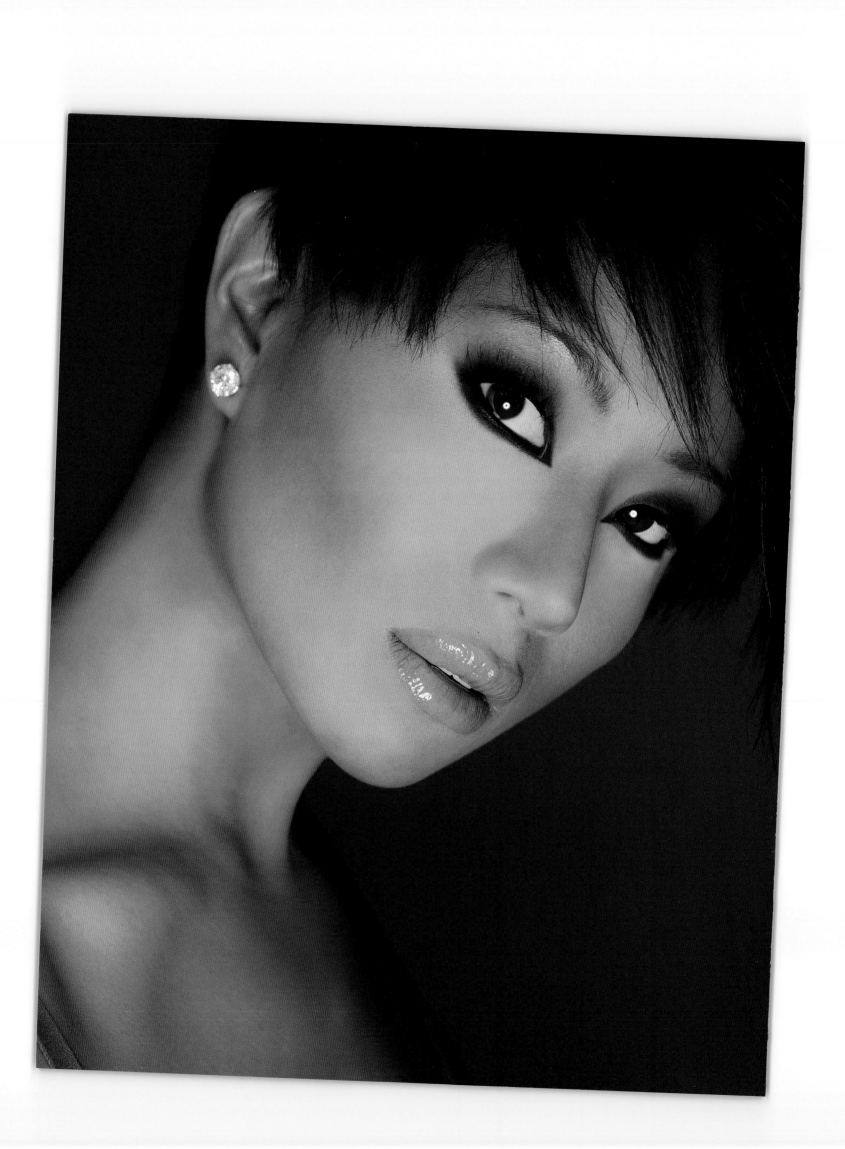

Danielle:
Shifting from Conservative to High-Impact

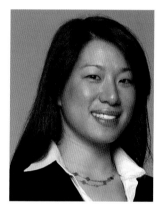

It would be easy to label Danielle as conservative. She graduated with a finance degree from Cornell University and now works for Bank of America. She's married and has two dogs (a miniature pinscher and a Brussels griffin) and does "adult things" on the weekends with her husband. But I only had to scratch the surface to discover that Danielle is anything but conventional. She has traveled to numerous countries, she's a serious hiker, and she climbs mountains—quite literally, having already scaled Mount Kilimanjaro. In addition to working long hours, she stays active playing tennis, going biking, or rollerblading. Next year, she plans to run the Chicago Marathon, simply because "it helps me to have a goal for physical fitness."

Danielle's a smart, fast-moving woman, and there's nothing stuffy or cautious about her—except her appearance. Her moderate, tailored look doesn't match her adventurous, goal-driven personality. It was time to update her look. Always open to something new and different, Danielle courageously took the plunge. Danielle's new look had such dramatic impact that even her husband barely recognized her.

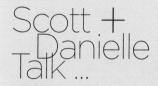

SCOTT: What is your typical beauty routine?
DANIELLE: I'm pretty basic. I don't really have a beauty routine. I usually get up late and roll out to work in about twenty minutes. So, that time consists of taking a shower, washing my face, putting on moisturizer with some protection, powder, mascara, and that's it. Oh, and usually some Chapstick. Today I actually put on some blush because I was concerned about my "before" shot. But in general, I'd say that I don't like to spend a lot of time focusing on me.

SCOTT: How about at night?
DANIELLE: I usually take a shower, wash my face, and then use a different moisturizer, a heavy night cream. No eye cream yet, although I'm told I'm supposed to start doing that. They say you're supposed to do it before you need it.

SCOTT: Are there things about yourself you wish you could change?

(continued on page 215)

Creating Danielle's Look

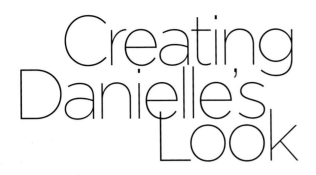

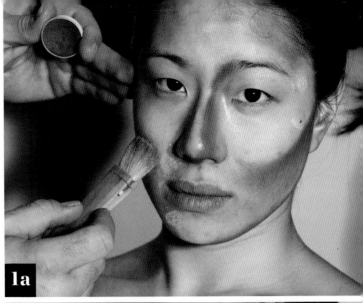

1a

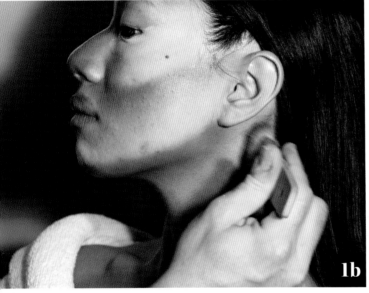

1b

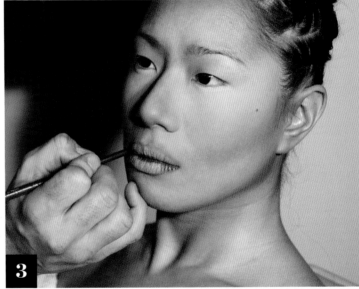

3

Tip Squint when looking at Danielle's contouring photo to better see the dark and light areas on her face.

Tip Be careful not to overdo the lining in the center of the bottom lip; otherwise, you'll make the lower lip look too small. You still want the lips to look as full and voluptuous as possible, but balanced.

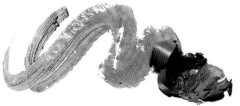

Daniel has a lovely oval face with pretty eyes and a beautiful nose and mouth. But she's faced with the same challenges many Asian women deal with: small eyes and no cheekbones. The trick to accentuating these features is to contour the face and elongate the eyes.

(continued from page 213)

1 Contouring, highlighting, and foundation

Most Asian faces are flatter planes. So, with Danielle, I needed to create sharper angles and "pop out the bones" with contouring and highlighting. *Remember: Keep in mind this rule of thumb when contouring and highlighting: Light adds, and dark takes away.* **(a)** Using light strokes with a goat hair brush, I applied contouring (dark) foundation: • Underneath the jaw line • Underneath the cheekbones • On the sides of the nose • At the inner eye where the bridge of the nose meets the brow bone • At the temples • Under the tip of the nose (gives the illusion of shortening the nose) **(b)** With shorter brushstrokes, I used a concealer brush to apply highlighting (light) concealer: • On top of the cheekbones • Underneath the eyebrows • On the bridge of the nose • At the center of the chin *Remember: When highlighting, try to put the lighter color where the sun might hit your face. Lightening these areas helps to draw the eye to these parts of your face.* **(c)** Using a separate goat hair brush, I applied a thin layer of warm beige cream foundation, moving the brush in small circles to delicately blend on top of the contouring and highlighting.

2 Cheeks

I used peachy-pink cream blush for Danielle's cheeks. This color, added some vibrancy to her cheeks. **(a)** I put a dab of cream blush on my finger and applied it to the apples of her cheeks. **(b)** I then used the foundation brush to blend it in, moving in a circular motion for a seamless transition between foundation and blush.

3 Lips

Danielle has a nice full lower lip. But it seemed to overpower her top lip, so I wanted to balance lower with upper. I used more muted colors so that the primary focus would remain on her eyes. **(a)** I followed the border of Danielle's upper lip with a dusty rose pencil. **(b)** I applied this same lip color to the inside center of her lower lip. This trick creates the illusion that the mouth is open, even when it's closed—pretty sexy, right? It also helps minimize the bottom lip, so it looks more balanced. **(c)** I finished off with a fleshy-colored sheer gloss.

DANIELLE: Probably if there was something I wish I could change about my look, I'd rather have glowing skin. I don't have great skin, by any means. It's something I've never had, so yeah, I'd love to have great, flawless, glowing skin. Something I feel has always made me different is my eyes. And my lips—I have fuller lips. So, these are things I've grown to appreciate about my face.

SCOTT: Do you have a certain idea of what "beautiful" is to you?
DANIELLE: I think beauty is something timeless, natural. I believe there's something attractive in everyone. I think it's about finding a way to highlight whatever that something is. So, perhaps beautiful is about finding your uniqueness.

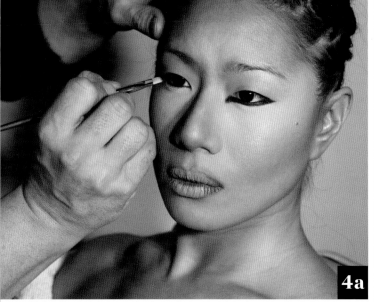

4a

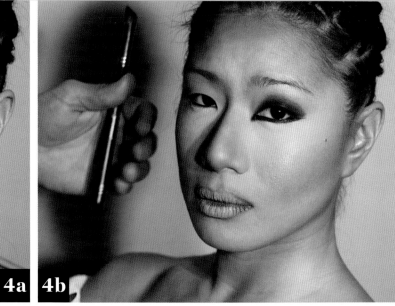

4b

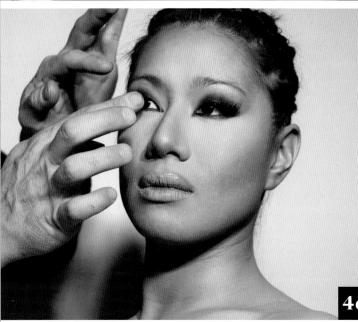

4c

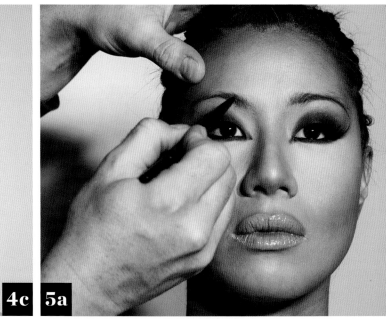

5a

Tip When filling in eyebrows, always follow your brow bone. And if you extend your eyeliner on your eye, be sure to also extend the eyebrow tail the same length so the brow doesn't stop short.

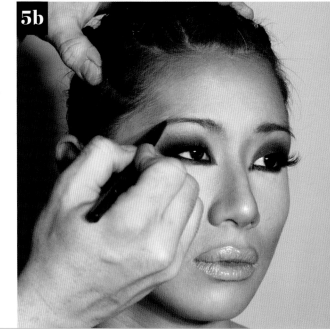

5b

4 Eyes

To give the illusion of a larger eye, I elongated the length of the Danielle's eyes in both directions to give her eyes more magnetism. **(a)** With a black eyeliner pencil, I lined her whole eye, making sure to extend the inner corner and outer corner of the eye. **(b)** With a medium eye shadow brush, I applied a black eye shadow and kept blending it out to create more width and depth. In general, the more you blend, the softer the effect. **(c)** I finished off with a demi lash on the outside corner of her eye. Demi lashes are better than full lashes for Asian eyes, because if you put eyelashes in the inner corners, it has a tendency to make the eyes look too close together.

5 Eyebrows

Asian eyebrows have a tendency to grow straight out, so it sometimes looks like the eyebrows are unruly. Danielle has well-shaped eyebrows naturally, so it was more about filling them in and getting them to lie flat than about reshaping them. **(a)** I did some minimal trimming with the razor comb and plucked a stray hair or two to flatten the brows. **(b)** I filled in the brow with a light brown eyebrow pencil. The wax from the pencil helps smooth down the hairs. Also, the darker hairs in the brow already create enough depth, so filling in with a lighter color still results in a dark eyebrow without the eyebrow appearing too overdrawn, as it would with a darker eyebrow pencil color.

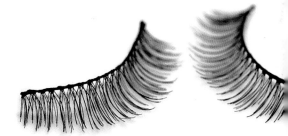

Tip To create a demi lash, simply cut a regular pair of false eyelashes in half. Then be sure to use the outside half of the lash for the outside corner of the eye. You can also double up these two halves and place one on top of the other for one thick demi lash for added drama.

REACTIONS...

Danielle's Reaction to Her Transformation

"Scott did things I never would've done to myself because I never would've even known to try them. Like the dramatic eye colors. I think maybe one of the reasons why my daily look is so plain is because I've never experimented with my eyes. I also had no idea that the contouring of the cheeks could have such a dramatic result. I would definitely do this for an evening event when I want more impact. I had been considering changing the shape of my eyebrows—going to an eyebrow specialist—because they can change your face. But Scott didn't really do anything to them

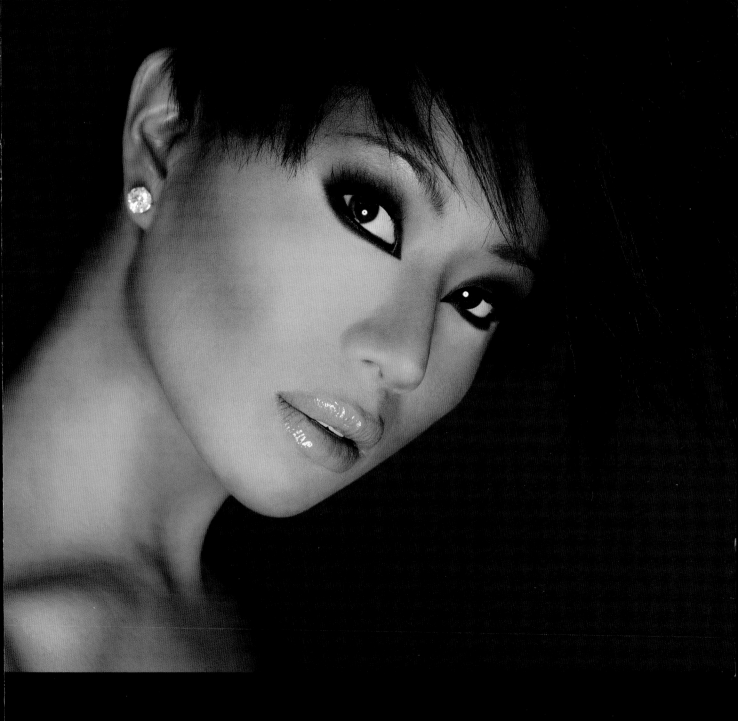

beyond minimal trimming and applying makeup, yet suddenly I really love the way they look. They really seem to fit my face just from the subtle changes in makeup."

"The experience has definitely given me a different sense of confidence. It's almost surreal to see how I was before. I feel like my regular look is no longer adequate. It's like I'm a totally different person. I think this is the most beautiful I've ever been in my entire life!"

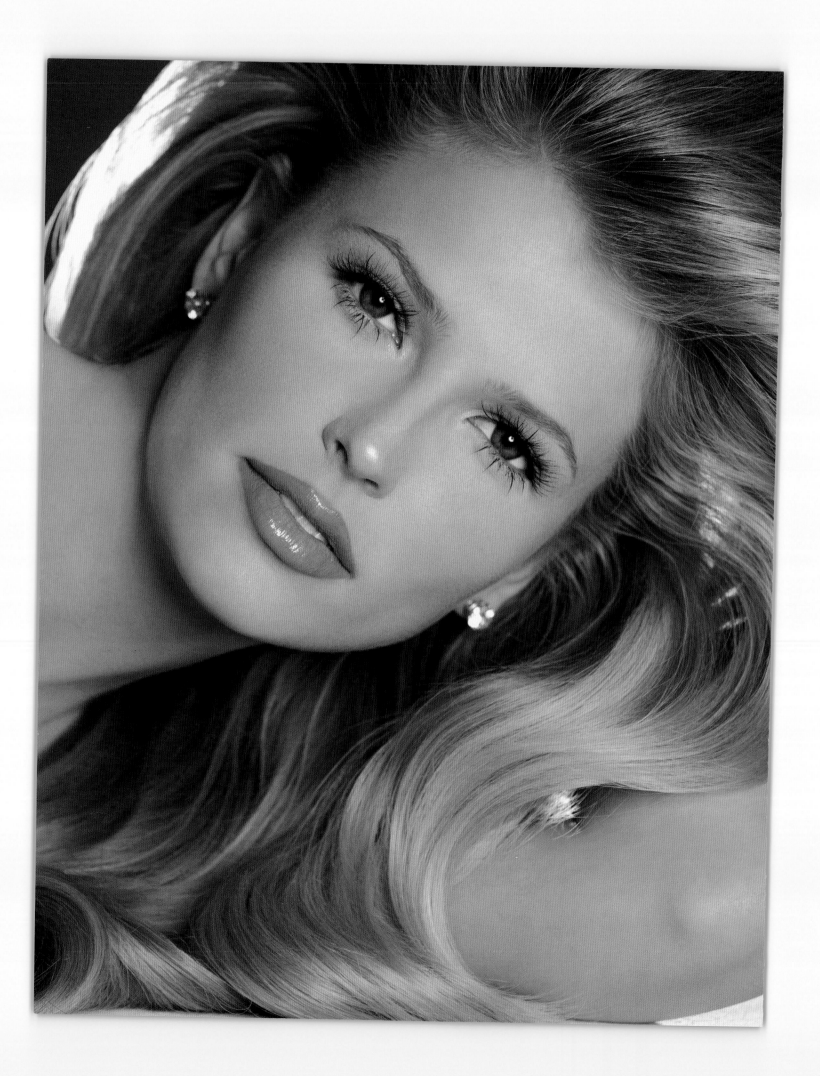

Lauren:
Blending Cooler Tones for More Sizzle and Pop

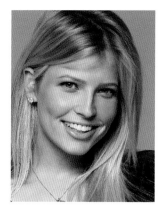

Here's my twist on a classic American beauty. Born in Champagne, Illinois, Lauren has a sunny look and demeanor that make her the perfect model for clients who want the wholesome, girl-next-door or bride-to-be type. While not dissatisfied with her look (she works all the time), Lauren expressed interest in taking a new direction. Without drastically changing her look, I wanted to unearth a more timeless beauty, more reminiscent of a Catherine Deneuve. With her transformation, we took Lauren from Champagne, Illinois, to Champagne, France, the birthplace of sparkling white wine.

Scott + Lauren Talk ...

SCOTT: In the morning when you get up, what do you do?

LAUREN: I wash my face and I put on a tinted sunscreen with an SPF of 15 or 30. That's pretty much it for the morning. If I have to put on makeup, I use some tinted moisturizer, concealer, sometimes mascara, and blush.

SCOTT: How about at the end of the day?

LAUREN: At night I'm stricter. I always cleanse, and use toner and moisturizer; I put a lot of moisturizer on my eyes. I also try to drink a lot of water before I go to bed. I try to drink two liters a day. I notice a difference in my skin with traveling on planes all the time. The water helps a lot.

(continued on page 223)

Creating, Lauren's Look

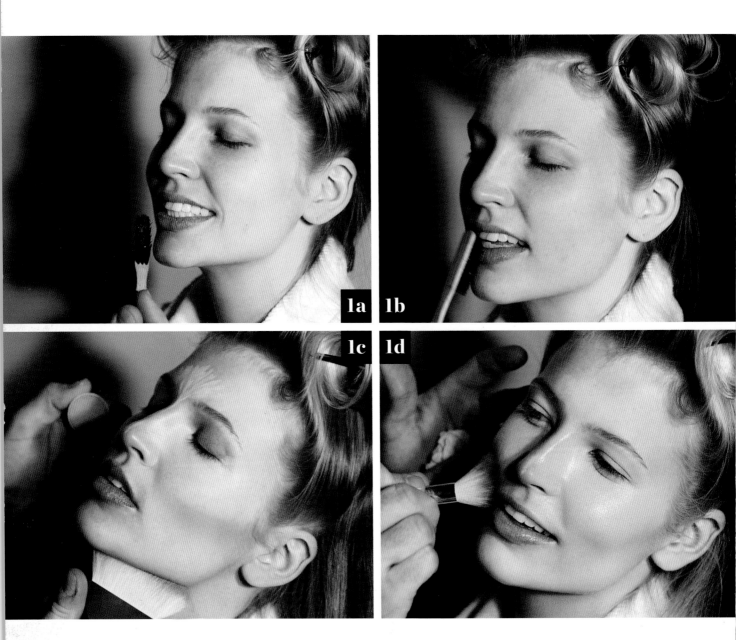

1a 1b
1c 1d

With Lauren, I wanted to shift the focus from her smile to her eyes, which tended to get lost. Lauren has hooded eyes, and it can be challenging to make hooded eyes appear more open. With her fair coloring, I knew I couldn't put a lot of additional color on her face. I also knew that shifting her coloring from warmer tones to cooler, icy tones would help accentuate her piercing blue eyes.

1 Contouring, highlighting, and foundation

I cooled down Lauren's skin using a foundation that didn't have a lot of yellow tone in it, which tends to give a warmer look. Instead, I used a very cool neutral (a beige-pink tone). A cooler, "icier" foundation with blue in it allowed the skin to reflect back into the cool blue of her eyes for more depth. And when I say "blue," I mean a very subtle undertone; we weren't trying to create a Smurfette! **(a)** Using light strokes with a goat hair brush, I applied contouring (dark) foundation: • Underneath the jaw line • Underneath the cheekbones **(b)** With short brush strokes, I used a concealer brush to apply highlighting (light) concealer: • Under the eyes • On top of the cheekbones • Underneath the eyebrows • On the bridge of the nose • At the center of the chin **(c)** Using a separate goat hair brush, I applied a thin layer of cooler beige-pink cream foundation on top of the contouring and highlighting and blended thoroughly, marrying all the colors together for a seamless transition between colors.

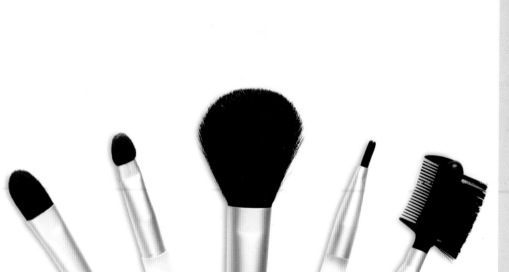

(continued from page 221)

SCOTT: What would you say is the most important thing for staying beautiful?
LAUREN: Exercise. I always exercise. For a while it was cardio and weight training, but now I'm doing more cardio and Pilates. I do a class here in New York that's all isometrics at a ballet bar—it's Pilates that incorporates natural body movements. All lengthening and strengthening, that's my favorite.

SCOTT: Are there models you admire?
LAUREN: Yes, Cindy Crawford and Heidi Klum. I think they're two women who have set great examples for what modeling can be. They've got great careers, and they balance them with an incredibly strong family life, which is really important to me. They also have maintained really wholesome images, which I admire. So, they've found a way to have the whole package.

(continued on page 225)

Remember, half of feeling good is looking good, and looking good leads to **FEELING GOOD.**

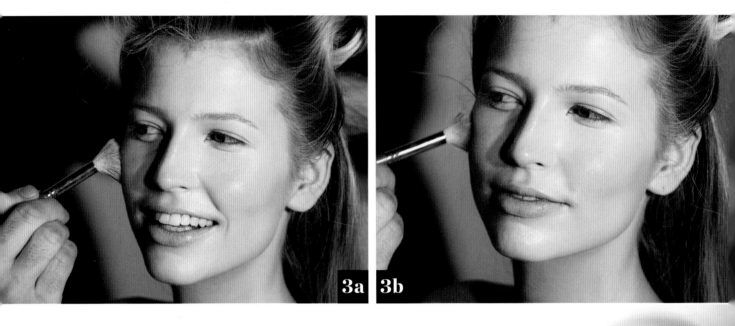

3a   3b

Tip Make sure to keep the highlighter on the apples of your cheeks; otherwise, your skin will look greasy. It's called a highlighter for a reason. Use it to hit the high points on your face.

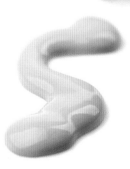

2 Eyes

Lauren has a dark blue ring around the outside of her iris, which was hard to see. While the cooler foundation helped to wake up the blue in Lauren's eyes, I knew we could open them up even more. But I also knew I would have to use minimal eye shadow, since Lauren has a hooded eye. Heavy color would only result in minimizing her eyes. What little color I did use was a very, very pale gray, a color I call Cashmere, which provides very soft, subtle shading. **(a)** I asked Lauren to keep her eye open and look straight ahead. Using a soft brush, I placed the Cashmere eye shadow directly above where the eye was open. This creates a color wash and provides a bit of depth without adding a lot of color. Think: creating a "shadow" in the eye. **(b)** I curled her eyelashes with an eyelash curler. **(c)** I applied a thin coat of black mascara. **(d)** I applied individual false eyelashes. I used three different lengths of lashes to create a kind of starburst effect. This helps keep the eye airy and open. A heavy lash would have the effect of closing up the eye. *Remember: Placement of individual false eyelashes is key. Putting the lashes on the outside corner keeps the eye more open and pulls the eye out from the center of the face. Putting the lashes on the inside of the eye, on the other hand, gives a more doe-eyed appearance.*

3 Cheeks

Instead of using a blush, I used a champagne shimmer highlighter on the apples of Lauren's cheeks. I didn't want to introduce pink into the skin because I wanted the skin to remain a cool tone.

(continued from page 223)

SCOTT: Do you think women spend too much time on their appearance?
LAUREN: In one sense, it's so great to be able to express yourself physically and have fun with makeup and show how great you can look. But I do think sometimes that women might take it a little too far. They don't fully appreciate the way they are, and they all start trying to look the same. I really believe that each of us is special. I think it'd be nice if everyone could embrace what they have and play with what they have. For example, I've always wanted to be really, really tan, but I'm not. I'm Swedish and I'm light, so I embrace that.

SCOTT: Is there something about yourself that you're most proud of?
LAUREN: I like my skin, probably because I've taken good care of it. Growing up in Florida, I was always out in the sun. And my dad, a doctor, would always say, "Sunscreen, sunscreen, sunscreen," when my girlfriends were going to tanning spas and lying out. So, I was pretty strict with myself.

(continued on page 227)

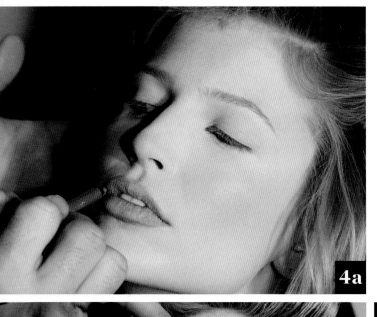

4a

Cooler, icey tones would help accentuate her piercing blue eyes.

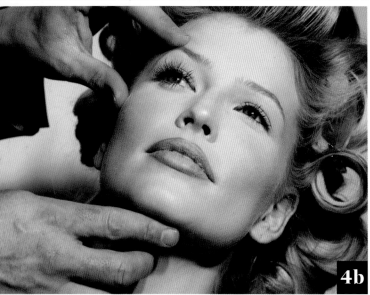

4b

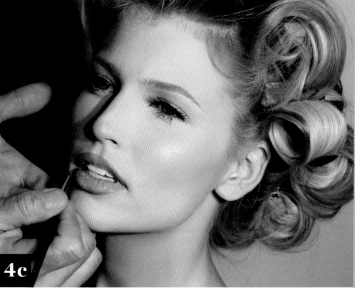

4c

Tip Brushing dry lips also gets the blood flowing, which makes your lips look fuller with more color!

(continued from page 225)

4 Lips

Before applying any lip color, I showed Lauren how she could smooth out dry, chapped lips by using a lip balm and a boar's hair brush. (You can find a natural bristle brush at your local health food store. A plastic toothbrush is too abrasive on your lips.) I scrubbed the lips back and forth to gently exfoliate and slough off the dead skin. I wanted to balance Lauren's upper lip with her bottom lip since she has a thinner upper lip. But I didn't want to minimize the bottom lip, as I did with Danielle. I wanted to enhance her top lip. So, I filled out her top lip with a trick I call "connecting the twin peaks." **(1)** With a lip liner that matched her natural lip color, I lightly connected the two highest points ("twin peaks") on Lauren's upper lip to give the illusion of more fullness. **(2)** I filled in the rest of the lip with a beige full-coverage lip gloss to complete the look.

5 Setting the look

I finished off with a nice dusting of translucent powder so as not to change the color of the foundation and the blush.

Tip To create more fullness in the top lip without overlining, lightly connect over the peaks with a natural-colored lip liner. This gives the illusion of a more pouty lip and is a nice update to the old "cupid bow" lips.

SCOTT: What are you least proud of?
LAUREN: Well, one thing I don't like about myself is that I have to work out so hard, so often. Food is my biggest battle. I love food, but it conflicts with my career. I try to eat a lot of fruits and vegetables and protein, but I still eat the things I want to eat, including things that are not good for me, like margaritas and quesos. That means I have to work out a lot—every day, for one to two hours.

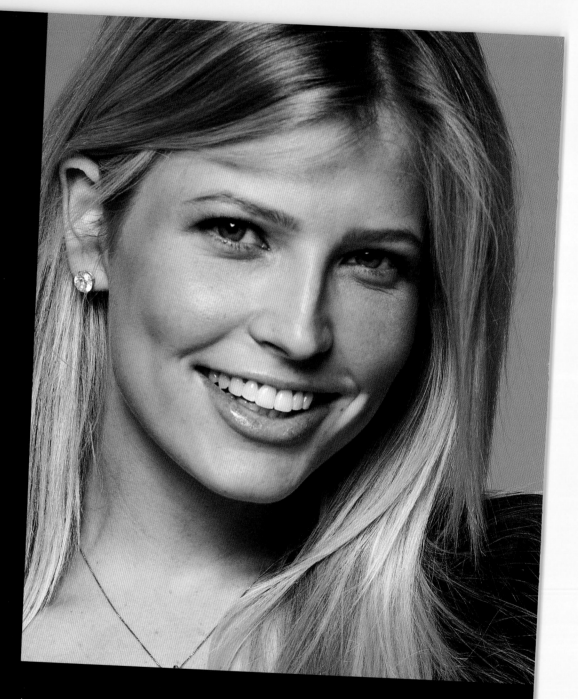

REACTIONS...

Lauren's Reaction to Her Transformation

"My skin looked like porcelain! I've always had the clean, fresh look for shoots like bridal stories, but nothing like what Scott did with the grays and cooler colors. I've always tried to enhance my eyes, bring out the blue, and always try to make my skin look dewy and fresh, but I've never tried using anything but warm colors. It's amazing the difference a cooler shade can make."

"The other thing was the eyelashes...I really want to get good with false eyelashes because they really opened up my eyes and added

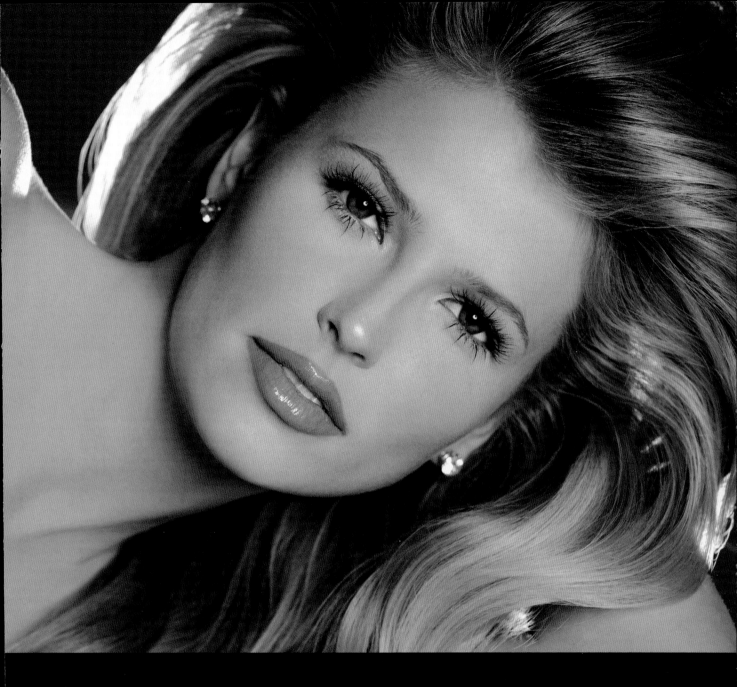

a kind of sparkle. The other great trick I now use is drawing the line on top, straight across, on my upper lip. It definitely makes my lips look fuller."

"I'm excited to have learned how to create a new look. It's so easy to get stuck in what I find comfortable and what I know looks okay. So I don't experiment. It was really nice to learn how to do something so glamorous for a change."

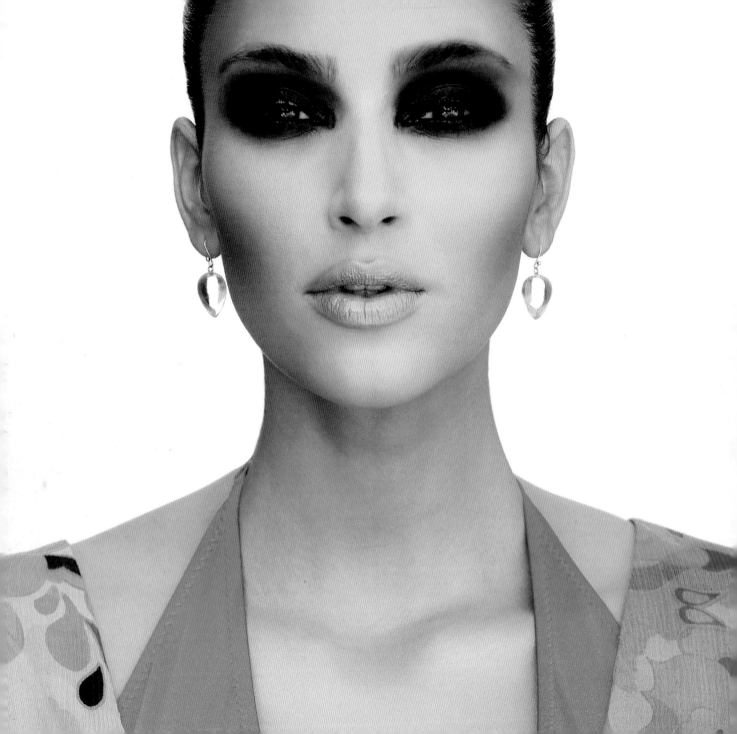

Kim Kardashian ★

Scott on Kim

Kim and I had never met before her transformation, but I knew she was a very pretty woman. I soon discovered upon meeting Kim that she is also very intelligent. She has an entrepreneurial spirit and seems to know how to turn any situation to her advantage—in a way that shows she inherently understands the awesome power and necessity of marketing in the world of showbiz, which is amazing considering she's still so young and relatively new to the business. We saw her in action when she intentionally left our studio sporting a blonde wig without letting on that it was just that—a wig. She knew going from brunette to blonde would work the paparazzi into a lather. And sure enough, she had the talk shows and the tabloids buzzing about her "new look." Kim waited two days before finally revealing that she was wearing a wig, which of course created another flurry of excitement. Like I said, she intrinsically gets it.

If that isn't impressive enough, Kim is also hard-working. She starts her day at 5:00 a.m. so that she can get in a workout before moving on to manage her various businesses. And the best part? With all she has going on, Kim still maintains a positive and energetic spirit. She has this amazing way of lighting up a room that makes everyone around her feel positive and happy, just like she is. It's no wonder she's been so successful.

Physically, Kim is freakily symmetrical. Is it fair to say hers is one of the prettiest faces I've worked on? No, it's not. I've worked with too many gorgeous women, all beautifully unique. But I can say Kim is the prettiest Armenian woman I've transformed. (Okay, she's also my first.) She can wear any look, so I decided to take her from Hollywood celebrity to fashion model. It's not every day that she gets to be so pa-pow! So, why not? After all, she can rival any supermodel, complete with curves that make her that much more luscious.

Physically, Kim is freakily SYMMETRICAL.

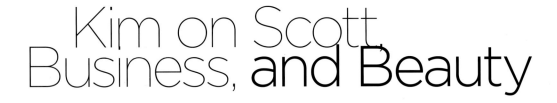

Kim on Scott,
Business, **and Beauty**

I have several things going now: my own perfume, a workout DVD, and a shoe line called ShoeDazzle.com, which basically offers a person their own shoe stylist who helps pick out a pair of shoes.

I also spend time working with The Dream Foundation, an organization that grants wishes to terminally ill adults. This is a cause that's very close to my heart. I attend events, and sometimes I help to fulfill a person's dream. For example, an adult might have a last wish to meet a celebrity or go to a sporting event. There was one girl who just wanted to get her hair and makeup done and spend the day with me, so that's what we did: spent the day together. We had an amazing time. She wrote me a beautiful letter before she died, which was very fulfilling for me too.

People ask whether I find it depressing. I don't, although there can be a huge element of sadness. My dad obviously passed away as an adult, and if he were to have a last wish, I would've liked to have granted that for him. So, now I'm helping other people by helping them ease their last few months or weeks. Overall, I'd say it's more heartwarming than depressing. I just always try to look at the positive side of things: A person got his or her final wish granted, and I was able to help with that.

Staying positive and feeling good is important in life and is a huge part of feeling beautiful. I'm definitely an advocate of taking care of oneself when it comes to beauty. I blog about it all the time. I am not a big drinker, and I definitely go to lots of events. But I'm extremely focused, and I sleep. Sleep is so important and is probably the main reason why I have so much energy. I also make sure I exercise every day, drink water, and take care of myself in general. I work out

in the morning—you just have to make time for it. I think it's really about making a commitment to yourself.

It's also important not to pay too much attention to what's in the magazines, their beauty standards, because there are so many different kinds of beauty. I'm very curvy, not your stick-skinny Hollywood girl, and I'll never be that tall, skinny supermodel; that's just not me. But I've learned to embrace who I am, embrace my shape. Everyone should try to do what they can to work with what they've got. I think if everyone did that, they'd be a lot happier. Why waste all that time worrying about things you can't change? I believe everyone can be happy, but you've got to do what it takes to look your best. Then you'll feel your best. That's just how it works!

Our deepest fear is not
that we are inadequate.
Our deepest fear is that
we are powerful beyond measure.
It is our light, not our darkness,
that most frightens us.
We ask ourselves, who am I to be brilliant,
gorgeous, talented, and fabulous?
Actually, who are you not to be?

—Nelson Mandela

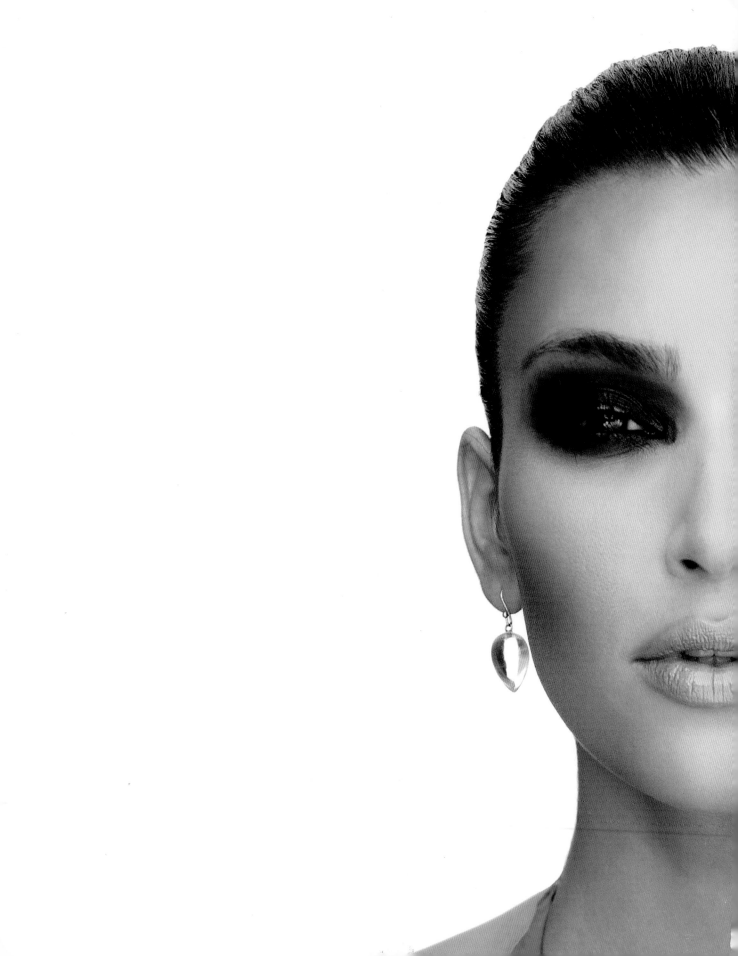

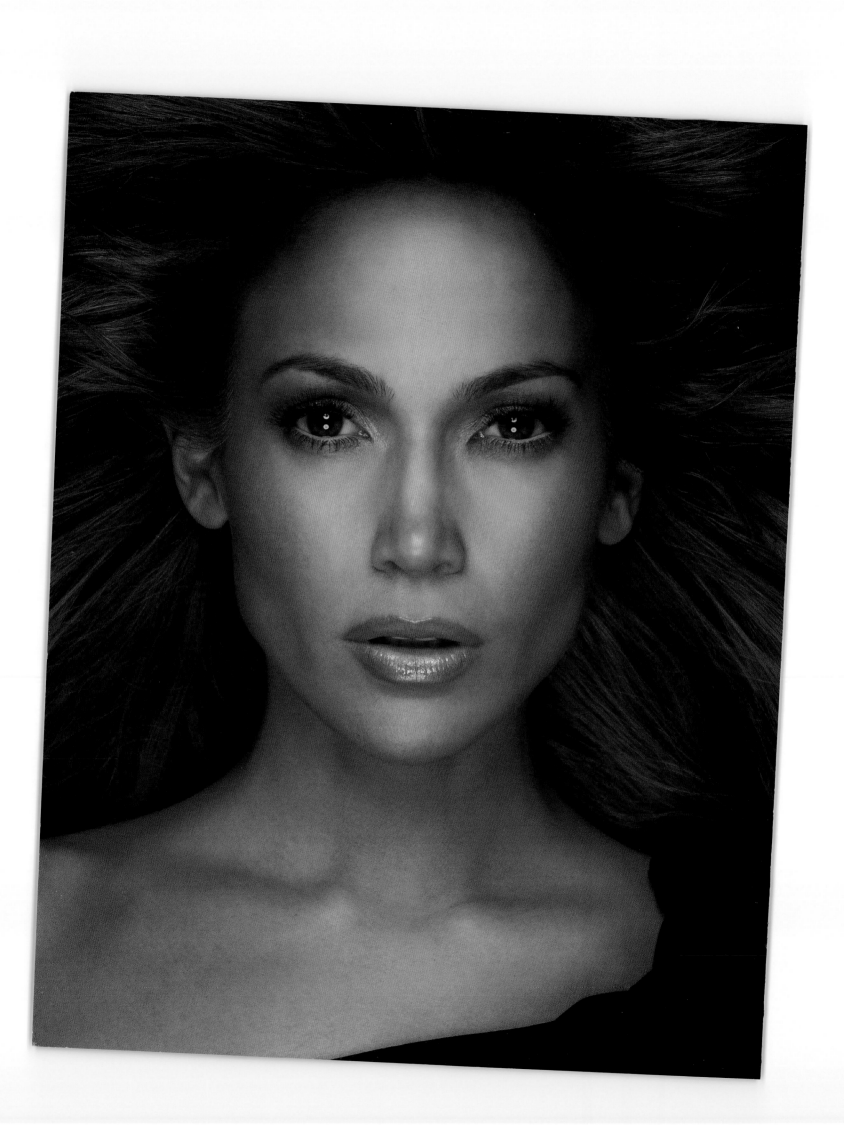

From Scott

The first time I laid eyes on Jennifer Lopez she was wearing a pair of jeans, high heels, a blue leather jacket, a turtleneck, and a pair of blue aviators. Her hair was pulled back and she was wearing no makeup. She looked radiant.

Up to this point, I had seen Jennifer with a certain "look." She was always made up to project structure, with lots of contour and shading. But for this photo shoot, I wanted her to look like herself, just the best possible version of that. She sat down and I began a series of beauty rituals to tap into her essence and to release what was already there but was waiting to come out. Halfway through our session, Jennifer started to radiate. She began to notice her reflection in the mirror. The results were extraordinary.

That same day Jennifer asked me to do her makeup for her *J.Lo* album cover, and we've been working together ever since. For the first two years, we maintained a monochromatic look, establishing her as a glowing bronze beauty. I created an entire movement from working with J. Lo, and suddenly, being the fashion icon that she is, bronze skin, beige lips, and a monochromatic palette was the new look. Jennifer became recognized as one of the most beautiful women in the world.

Jennifer connected with her inner beauty. And I believe every woman has the potential to do the same. Jennifer and I have taught each other many things. She's been a positive presence in my life ever since the day we met. I will always be grateful for that.

Scott

About the Author

Scott Barnes is a celebrated makeup artist and innovator within the cosmetics industry.

He arrived in New York City in 1984 determined to fulfill his dream as a fine-arts painter. After attending New York's prestigious Parsons School of Design, Scott began assisting on fashion photography shoots and quickly became one of the most sought after makeup artists in the industry.

International beauty guru Shu Uemura selected Scott to revamp his Atelier Made line, which became a huge success within the fashion industry and among celebrities. Following his success at Shu Uemura, Scott launched his own twenty-one-piece color cosmetic line, Scott Barnes Cosmetics, on QVC in April 2004. Five months later, Scott introduced 130 products at Holt Renfrew, in Canada, Saks Fifth Avenue, in the U.S., and other high-end specialty boutiques. A year later, the collection launched in Europe and Australia and became an overnight success for which *Women's Wear Daily* named Scott the "Newcomer of the Year." He was also a finalist for the Fashion Group International's "Rising Star" award.

Scott Barnes has worked with world-renowned photographers, including Patrick Demarchelier, Scavullo, Gilles Bensimon, Tony Duran, Peter Lindbergh, Annie Leibovitz, Ruven Afanador, and Mark Seliger with his work gracing the covers of such leading magazines as *Allure, Elle, Harper's Bazaar, InStyle, Vanity Fair, Rolling Stone*, and *Marie Claire*. Scott has also appeared on top national and regional television programs, such as *The Oprah Winfrey Show, Extra, Access Hollywood*, and *Good Day L.A.*

Although Scott has worked with a variety of Hollywood talent over the years, including Kate Hudson, Beyonce, Gwyneth Paltrow, and Celine Dion, it's his work with Jennifer Lopez that birthed the new monochromatic look featuring bronzed skin and pale lips. Described as "The Glow," this signature look became known as "lit from within" and helped launch Scott's best-selling beauty product, Body Bling bronzer.

In addition to numerous ad campaigns and music videos, Scott's work on set includes such films as *El Cantante*, which earned him Oscar consideration. Scott was also responsible for Jennifer Lopez's memorable Cinderella moments in *Maid in Manhattan*.

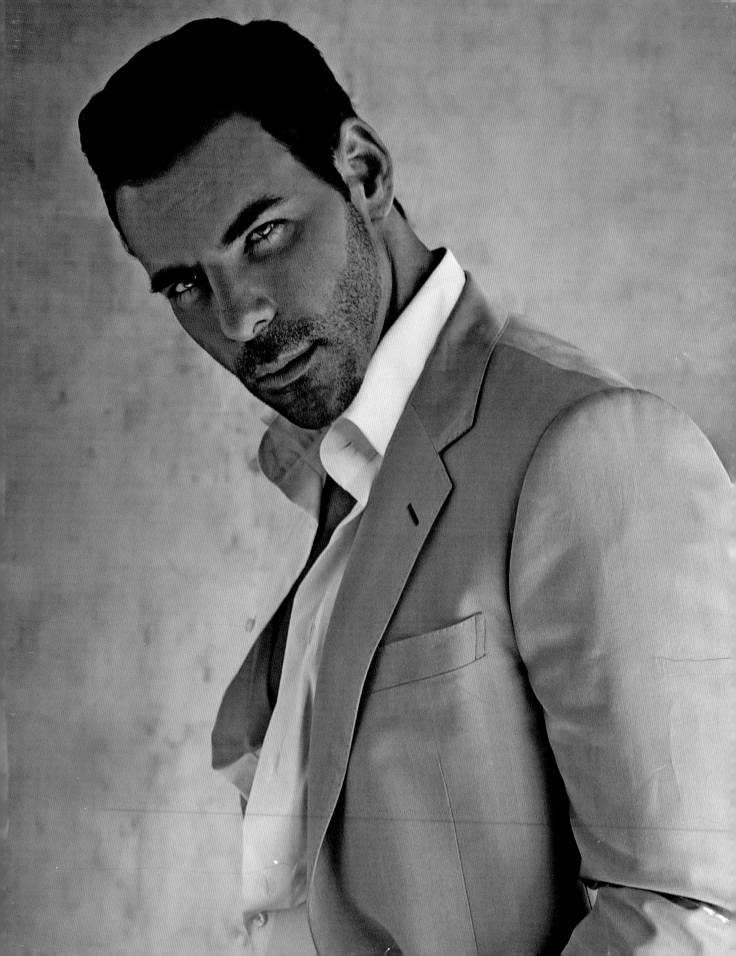

Acknowledgments

Making this book has been a huge undertaking and a testament to my faith. I would like to thank God for his steadfast love, thank you!

I would like to thank the following people for all their hard work and dedication:

Fair Winds Press for the opportunity and belief in this book. Will Kiester, Rosalind Wanke, and Sylvia McArdle, thank you for making this a great experience. I would like to thank David D'Amico, you were a godsend, I would love to do it again. Lydia Latrowski, you keep me looking smooth. Jennifer Lopez and Mark Anthony, Simon Fields, Debbie Izzard, Celine Dion. Karl Simone, who has always been a great friend and a wonderful photographer. Jocelyn Goldstein, for her fly sense of style. Chuck "Chuckie Love" Amos, make it bigger, wilder, and sexier! Dana Benningfield, you took all my words and made sense of them, Phew…! Lorraine Schwartz, for your stunning jewelry. Lenny and Antonia Trimarchi, your jewelry "rocks." Larry Schatz, for your constant belief in me, what can I say, I am blessed to have you on my side. Milk Studios, for a beautiful workspace to create beauty. Oscar Reyes and Dani Bongiorno. Kim Kardashian, Judith Light, Mariska Hargitay, and Kat Deluna. Dr. Jessica Wu, I told you!!! Dr. Eva Cwynar, Maureen and Marley Kornowa, thank you for sharing your story with us, it means the world to me. Diane Von Furstenberg, Michael Kors, Catherine Malandrino, Marc Jacobs, and everyone else who assisted me on these shoots. And my Family, especially my Godmother, Aunt Jackie, whose unwavering support pushed me to be my best.